The Stress Mess

—

How to Thrive
in Turbulent Times

The Stress Mess

How to Thrive
in Turbulent Times

Kelsie Kenefick

Roots and Wings Publishing

First edition – First printing
Printed in the United States

ISBN 978-0977749317

Library of Congress Card Number: 2008941684

Cover design by Bill Hubschwerlin
Interior design by Kay Turnbaugh
Photography by Tom Rampton
Illustrations by Bill Hubschwerlin

Disclaimer: The author of this book recommends that all persons with physical or mental symptoms of stress see their doctor for an accurate diagnosis before beginning this program. This book is meant to be used in conjunction with your doctor's supervision. The author and publisher accept no legal responsibility for any actions that you may choose to take relating to matters contained in this book. This book is sold with the understanding that you are choosing to take responsibility for your well-being and for mastering the skills necessary to eliminate your stress induced symptoms.

Names and identifying details of all patients' stories have been changed to protect confidentiality.

To my mom and dad for giving me life

*To my spiritual teachers for teaching me how to celebrate life
and to live it with joy and grace*

*To the doctors in Colorado who believed in my work and sincerely wanted
to see their patients come to a place of living naturally pain free*

*To my patients throughout the years who were a delight and inspiration
to work with and taught me so much about everything*

Thank you

Acknowledgements

I have had the most amazing group of people around me support-ing the birth of this book. Without them this book would not be all that it is. It is with heartfelt gratitude that I say thanks to the following people.

Thank you Mary Anne Maier, editor, who who did a a fabulous job. Thank you to Bill Hubschwerlin who did both the book cover design and the beautiful illustrations in this book. Thank you to Tom Ramp-ton, author, photographer, and publisher, for the photographs used throughout the book. Thank you to Kay Turnbaugh for the interior design. Each was a true delight to work with and helped to make this a smooth process. I sincerely appreciate all of them for their professional work and their patience as I moved through the creation this book.

Thank you to the following people who did proofreading and com-menting at various stages during the book preparation process: Dr. Michele Fecteau (osteopathic physician); Gary Hannemann (licensed professional counselor); Colleen Kenefick (medical librarian, State Uni-versity of New York at Stony Brook); Evie Paur (biofeedback therapist, Boulder Community Hospital); and Alan Wright (dear friend). It is with love and deep appreciation that I say thank you to these special people for their proofreading, support, and encouragement.

Thank you to the Colorado Independent Publishers Association (CIPA) for teaching me all that I needed to know about book writing and publishing and for helping me to get my program into print so that many can benefit. Thank you to all of the volunteers in CIPA for donat-ing their time and creating a great organization.

Creating a book is a team effort, and I was blessed to have an amazing team. I appreciate each of these people for their unique contributions.

CONTENTS

Step 3 – Calm the Body/Still the Mind

Lesson 3 – *Breathing Your Way to Relaxation*

Lesson 4 – *Deep Relaxation of the Body-Mind*

Step 4 – Relax Specific Muscles

Step 5 – Tap into the Power of Your Mind

Step 6 – Increase Your Circulation

Lesson 11 – *Dilating Your Arteries for Deeper Relaxation*

Step 7 – Stay on Track

Lesson 12 – *Living Beyond the Stress Mess*

1

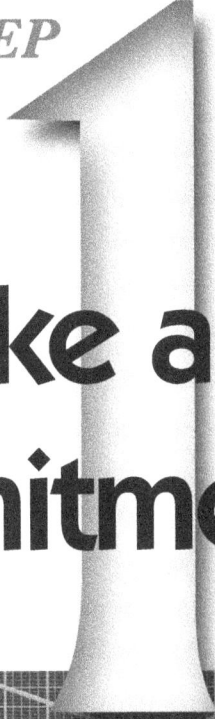

Make a
Commitment

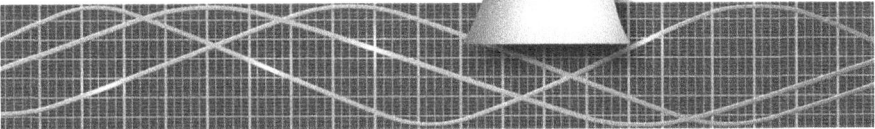

Introduction

The program presented in this book was carefully developed after years of successful work with patients in my clinical practice as a certified biofeedback therapist. It is with gratitude to my patients and to the doctors in Colorado who believed in my work that I am able to bring this program to you.

This book teaches you how to control symptoms which are either stress induced or exacerbated by stress. The following are just some of the physical and mental symptoms which were successfully brought under control with the techniques presented in this book: headaches, irritable bowel syndrome, anxiety, panic attacks, cancer pain & nausea from treatment, TMJ disorders, insomnia, high blood pressure, chronic pain, epileptic seizures, and fibromyalgia.

Your ability to control your stress response will be very empowering. Patients regularly report to me that they experience a sense of empowerment upon completing the steps of this process that carries over into many other areas of their lives. Once you realize just how much control you have over your physiology, you will begin to realize how much power you have in other areas of your life as well. If you can gain control over your stress, and the resulting physical and mental symptoms, imagine what else you can do in your life!

Congratulations to you for embarking upon this exciting and powerful journey. Your choice to move through this time of global turbulence with a clear mind and strong body will serve us all. My hope is that you enjoy the process as much as the results.

Deciding to Master Your Stress

Moving Beyond the Stress Mess— Getting Started

Do you feel anxious about the economy? Does your mind race out of control? Are you feeling like your stress has become unmanageable?

We are all going through enormous changes right now. Many of us who previously believed that we had control over our lives and destiny suddenly feel overwhelmed. With the uncertain economy and global changes affecting our jobs, homes, and even our ability to buy groceries, how can we manage to remain happy and healthy as individuals and in our relationships?

There are things we can control in life, others that we can at least influence, and still others that we have absolutely no control over. Especially in times of upheaval and uncertainty, it is helpful to identify those things we do have control over and build upon them. Making this our focus will help us stay positive and empowered through the changes and challenges we face.

Although many of us feel stress in reaction to these growing challenges, the good news is that we can actually take control of stress by choosing to take responsibility for it. Responsibility means "to respond with ability." Taking responsibility for our stress, or responding to it with ability, is very different from reacting to it. To react usually implies acting in opposition to something. Instead of having a knee-jerk reaction when we experience stress, we can learn to respond to it with calm and clear-headed awareness that keeps the stress within our control. .

You have probably heard that over 90 percent of doctor visits are "stress related." What does this mean? We certainly do not mean that stress is "all in your head." But you can be sure that if it is in your head, it will be in your body as well—and vice versa.

We've learned through research that when stress is left unchecked numerous damaging changes occur in both the body and the mind. We will look at many of these changes in chapter two. If the stress is not managed, it can lead to physical symptoms such as high blood pressure, headaches, backaches, irritable bowel syndrome, heart disease, and countless other symptoms. On the mental and emotional levels, unchecked stress can lead to insomnia, anxiety, panic attacks, inability to focus, and even violence.

Technological and medical advances have led us to believe in the possibility of quick fixes. We want to go to the doctor and have him or her fix us. But even if that were possible, by not participating in our own wellness, and instead relying solely on others to "fix us," we are giving our power away to them.

Learning to take control of your stress is a vital first step in taking that power back. While outside events over which you have no control may lead you to react with stress, the stress itself occurs within you and is also within your control. But to gain that control requires you to take a deep look within as a first step on your way to freeing yourself of the tension.

In becoming the master of your body and mind, you will be able to affect your reaction to external stressors. Typically, people let their minds control them instead of using the mind as the magnificent tool it can be when used properly. When you let your mind run rampant, you are likely to create unnecessary stress for yourself. Conversely, by learning to bring awareness to the mind, you can make constructive choices in response, rather than reaction, to external stressors.

The amount of stress people feel today is unprecedented. We're suddenly aware that we can no longer rely on external comforts to help us feel good. Many of us don't know how to cope with the magnitude of what is happening around us. Yet even amidst the major challenges we as individuals and our planet are facing, we can—and must—learn to calm the body and still the mind in order to think clearly and maintain our health.

With awareness you can bring yourself into balance. Eventually, perhaps the earth will come back into balance as well. But it is essential to begin with yourself. This book is not about changing external circumstances.

This program may seem too simple, at first, to have a dramatic impact on your life, but don't be deceived! Stick with it, even when you don't feel like doing it. You will find a sense of peace in your life when you learn to relax from within rather than counting on the external world to deliver the calm you're yearning for.

Are you ready to start on this great inward journey? Today is the day to begin learning to thrive from within—to move beyond the stress mess!

New Habits

This book is essentially about creating new habits. Did you know that everything you do in life is a habit? The new habits and skills you will bring into your life with this program will actually allow you to create a shift in your autonomic nervous system (ANS). This is the part of the nervous system that is not usually consciously controlled. What we think of as "automatic" functions, such as our blood flowing through arteries or our heart beating are regulated by the autonomic nervous system. Your ANS functions do occur automatically unless you consciously take control of them. When you have successfully made the proper shift in your autonomic nervous system by following the steps outlined here, and are able to maintain that shift, you will be able to control, or prevent, stress related symptoms.

The exercises in this program do not need to take a lot of your time every day. Eventually, you will have the skills well-integrated into your life, and you won't even need to set aside special time for practice. You will have created new habits. I have set up this process so that, even in the learning stages, it will take a minimal amount of time and still be effective.

Change does not always come easily, but you will find that the changes you make throughout this program are ones you will enjoy. These changes will leave you feeling stronger physically, mentally and emotionally. As your health, well-being and happiness grow, you will want these new habits to be a part of each day. They will become effortless.

Take a small sheet of paper now and write the following:

Everything I do is a habit.
I choose to create new habits.
I choose to be relaxed & at peace.

Now, place this reminder on your bathroom mirror, in your day planner or anywhere that it will help you remember this important point.

How to Use This Program Successfully

The steps for freeing yourself from the symptoms of stress have been set up in a specific order so that the skills build upon each other. You might think that controlling blood flow through your arteries is the most important part of the training and therefore feel tempted to skip right to that lesson. Don't do it! There are reasons why controlling blood flow is the last step in this program, just as there are reasons each step is included in the order it appears in the book. You will be much more effective learning each skill if you do it in this order. If you attempt to do the steps out of order, you may become frustrated when you find that you cannot do what you are being instructed to do or don't reach the level of success you had hoped for.

The program is divided into seven primary steps and 12 lessons supporting those steps. You will find the process most effective if you do one each week. There are two lessons that you will need a bit more time to work on: using your thoughts to heal (Lesson 10) and dilating your arteries (Lesson 11). Each lesson provides specific activities that you will need to practice daily. It is important to get into the habit of practicing and mastering one skill before moving on to a new one. Remember, you are forming new habits. Give yourself time for each new habit to take hold.

This is an *experiential* program—a program in which you make changes by participating in activities. At the end of each lesson, you will find a section titled "Practice" that contains a summary of what you will need to perform successfully before moving on to the next lesson. Reading the book without doing the exercises will not help significantly, if at all.

A Partner for Support

Many people find it helpful to have a partner for support when doing a program such as this. If you have a friend or relative with stress induced symptoms you might want to invite them to join you in doing this program. Moving through the program with another person can help both of you to stay on track and make the process more fun.

If you choose to move through this process with a partner, set aside a time once a week when you can check in and share your successes. This could be a phone date or you could get together in person. Be sure to decide each week which lesson(s) you will be doing during the following week.

The author of this book is available for coaching and support. For further information go to NaturallyStressFree.com and click on Consultations.

Staying on Track

You will find the changes you make in your life as you move through this book to be both enjoyable and empowering. People love integrating these positive new habits into their lives. Still, some people find themselves slipping back into old patterns at times. If you do get off track, simply be accepting of yourself and get back on track again.

Occasionally people will find themselves making excuses for why they go off track from the program. For example, they might say, "I am relaxed today, so I don't need to do it," or "I'm too busy today. I can't take the time to do it." If you find such thoughts filling your mind during the program, stop and notice the excuses running in your mind. Then, acknowledge what your mind is doing and say to yourself, "Thank you for sharing! I am going to complete this lesson and its practice steps anyway!"

Remember, everything is a habit. In creating new habits, you may experience some resistance at times. Be aware of the resistance, but do not let it stop you from moving forward.

This journey to a more relaxed life is about taking responsibility for your health, well-being and happiness. I have found that people with stress-induced physical symptoms are usually highly motivated and are very good at taking responsibility. By committing to this program, you are taking the empowering steps to creating a pain-free and more joy-filled life.

Many people find that a good way to develop these important new habits and stay on track is to work with the *The Stress Mess Workbook*. This hands-on workbook is a good reminder of the skills you need to practice daily and gives you forms for tracking your progress. All the worksheets and charts you need are included. You may purchase the workbook at the website listed at the bottom of the page.

Skeptical? The Program Will Work Anyway

It is okay to be skeptical! Perhaps you have suffered from an over-aroused nervous system for decades, and your mind simply cannot believe that you can control it. You may feel discouraged or feel like you have tried everything with little or no success. If you have not done this program, you have not tried everything. You can be successful with this program even if you are skeptical. My skeptics have always become my strongest supporters. You can notice your skepticism and acknowledge it. *Just don't let it stop you!*

I had one patient who suffered for more than 30 years from incapacitating migraines that she was having about three times a week. Her migraines made her completely nonfunctional. Mary* had tried many things over the decades—from herbs to acupuncture to chiropractic. She tried everything that anyone would suggest. Just before I saw her, Mary was going to the emergency room three times a week to get shots of morphine for her migraine headaches. As you may know, the more medication one takes the more tolerance the body builds up requiring higher and higher doses to achieve the same effect. One day Mary walked into the emergency room and said, "I need a higher dose of morphine; this isn't working anymore." At that point the doctors finally said, "If we give you a larger dose it will kill you. Why don't you try biofeedback?"

Mary came to me to learn the skills that you are about to learn in this book. Although skeptical, she was highly motivated. Mary was able to eliminate her muscle tension headaches in five sessions and her migraines in ten sessions. I tell people with migraines to plan on twelve to sixteen sessions to gain complete control of their migraines. When she got to the tenth session, Mary could not believe that her migraines were gone. Her mind had a hard time grasping this fact so she opted to do six more sessions. By the time she finished the training, her mind finally believed that it was true!

The program contained in this book will work whether or not you are skeptical of it. The key is to simply follow the program as it is set up, and you will be on your way to being healthier and more relaxed.

---

* Patients' names have been changed to protect their privacy

Working with Your Doctor

If you already have physical or mental stress induced symptoms an accurate diagnosis is medically essential. If you have high blood pressure, headaches, pain, IBS, depression, anxiety, panic attacks, insomnia, or any disorder caused, or exacerbated by stress please see your doctor. Furthermore, you need to have a doctor oversee the reduction of your medications as you move through this program, if that is appropriate to your situation.

If you do not currently have a doctor, you will want to find one who is caring and knowledgeable and who is compatible with you. Neurologists specialize in diseases that affect the brain and therefore are highly qualified to diagnose and treat headaches and other nervous system disorders. They tend to have a very good understanding of the autonomic nervous system and the use of biofeedback skills to make internal shifts. Osteopaths (D.O.s) also have a good understanding of the autonomic nervous system and the learned skills that can regulate it. Most neurologists and osteopath physicians will be able to support you through this program with understanding while overseeing your medication reduction.

If you have symptoms other than headache or a neurological disorder, find the appropriate doctor for your situation. When selecting a doctor to work with in this process, ask yourself the following questions:

- Does this doctor often treat people with my symptoms?

- Does he/she listen to me and take the time I need?

- Do I feel that I can talk honestly with this doctor without feeling that I am being judged?

- Is this doctor knowledgeable about using non-drug treatments like biofeedback for these symptoms?

Contraindications

Learning to make shifts in your nervous system to eliminate your stress induced symptoms will create changes in your body, mind and emotions. *The skills presented in this book should be considered contraindicated for the following disorders:*

- acute or fragile schizophrenia
- some paranoid disorders
- some dissociative disorders

If you have any questions about whether or not you should do this program consult your physician or a psychiatrist.

Declaring Your Commitment

Are you ready to make a commitment now to take control of your stress? Remember, you don't have to believe it; you just have to *do* it. You can choose to look forward to this program with excitement and a positive attitude. By making a commitment in writing, you strengthen your positive intention.

Write by hand the following statement:

I _____ (name) on this _____ day of _____, 20___, commit to the program, *Moving Beyond the Stress Mess*. I agree to follow the program as it is structured. I agree to have my doctor oversee the reduction of my medications, if applicable, as I move through this program. Finally, I declare that I am willing to create new habits.

Good! Now tape this declaration of your independence from stress to your refrigerator or somewhere you will see it every day.

If you want to give your intention and commitment even more power, speak them aloud to another person. You could voice your intent to your program partner, a significant other, a friend or relative. Tell them what you are going to do, what your intentions are and what your commitment is. Voicing your commitment out loud gives it strength. Let your word be law. Speak with power and affirmation

Practice

Below is a summary of activities to complete before moving on to the next lesson.

1. Put your commitment in writing and post it somewhere you will see it every day.

2. Find a partner to do the program with if you want this kind of mutual support.

3. Discuss this program with your doctor, if appropriate.

2

Understanding Stress

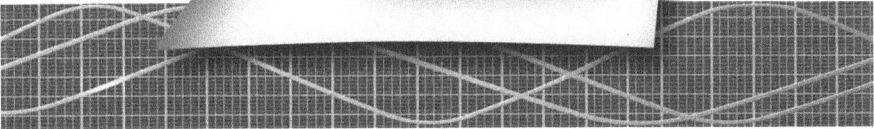

Knowing Your Body
And Tracking Your Progress

It is important to understand the physiology of stress before you move into the experiential activities contained in this book. You needn't comprehend this process in complex medical terms, but understanding it at a basic level is your first, essential step toward managing your nervous system and stress.

Stress Questionnaire

Begin by asking yourself the following questions regarding how your body and mind experience stress. Take out a sheet of paper and write down your answers. You may not currently have any physical symptoms resulting from stress. Simply answer the questions that are relevant to you and do the program anyway to prevent symptoms from occurring.

Stress Questionnaire

1. What mental or emotional symptoms of stress do you currently have? (i.e. anxiety, panic attacks, irritability, jumpiness, depression, etc)

2. What physical symptoms do you have that were created by stress or are made worse by stress? (i.e. high blood pressure, headaches, chronic pain, irritable bowel syndrome, TMJ disorder, fibromyalgia, insomnia, etc)

3. What have you done for your stress? What has worked? What hasn't worked?

4. Do you have pain or stiffness in your neck?

5. Do you have pain or stiffness in your shoulders?

6. Do you get headaches?

7. Do your teeth hurt? Do you clench or grind your teeth? Do you have a night guard to protect your teeth?

8. Do you ever get eyestrain (from computers, reading or other activities)?

9. Do you tend to have cold hands and feet?

10. Do you drink coffee or ingest any other caffeine (e.g., in tea or chocolate)?

11. Do you smoke cigarettes?

12. Do you feel overwhelmed?

13. Do you have thoughts of being violent towards yourself or others?

14. How would your life be different if you did not have physical, mental, or emotional symptoms of stress?

15. What would you like to achieve from doing this program? What are your goals?

Set your answers to these questions aside for now. We will be addressing several of these questions while reviewing the symptoms of stress later in this chapter. However, first it is important to understand the autonomic nervous system and its relationship to stress.

The Autonomic Nervous System

The nervous system has two main components. One part of it is consciously controlled while the other is usually not under voluntary control. If you want to lift your arm up, for example, you make a conscious decision to do so. The "autonomic" part of the nervous system, on the other hand, is the part that functions without thought, automatically.

You probably don't think about how blood flows through your arteries—it just flows! However, if you get migraine headaches or have high blood pressure, you can learn how to deliberately regulate vascular changes in the body (blood flow) to help control these problems. In the same way, you don't have to think about it to make your heart beat, but if you have a fast or irregular heart rate, you can learn how to stabilize it.

Other functions normally controlled by the autonomic nervous system are muscle tension, sweat gland activity, respiration and brain wave activity. We don't usually think about controlling these bodily functions because they do their jobs automatically. Most people don't even realize that it is possible to control such functions. The good news is that we *can* learn to control many physiological functions that affect symptoms by learning how to regulate this part of the nervous system.

The Fight-or-Flight Response

The ANS consists of two parts: the sympathetic nervous system and the para-sympathetic nervous system. In a nutshell, the sympathetic nervous system is associated with an aroused nervous system and the parasympathetic is associated with a normal level of tension in the body and the mind.

The sympathetic nervous system has only one job: to protect the body when there is a perceived threat or danger. The physiology to carry out this job developed in humans thousands of years ago. Early people had to protect themselves physically from lions, bears and other tribes, so it was critical that the body have strength and energy in an emergency. You may have heard of the term "fight or flight," which is how we describe this physiological response to danger. When threatened, the body gears up to fight and protect itself or to flee from the danger.

This mechanism still serves us today in crisis situations. For example, when you are driving in traffic, you may need to respond quickly to avoid an accident. If you needed to run into a burning house to save a loved one, your body would be charged up with strength and energy. You may have heard stories in which a mother is able to lift something as heavy as a car off her trapped child. Usually, a single woman or man would not have the strength to do that. But when the sympathetic nervous system is activated, the hormone called adrenaline is released into the bloodstream to give the body an extra boost of strength and energy.

I recall my second day of teaching high school in upstate New York. I was fresh out of college and was hired to teach a class of mentally, physically and emotionally handicapped teenagers and young adults. As I sat at my desk that morning, a young man walked into the room and put a knife to my throat. I felt the cold blade against my skin. Despite my terror, I looked up at him and told him to put the knife away. He started laughing! Little did I know that I had said the perfect thing. He thought it was very funny that I called it a knife and said, "It's not a knife–it's a switchblade!" Amidst his laughter and amusement that I didn't know the difference between a knife and a switchblade, he put the weapon away.

Think about how your body would react, as mine did that day, if someone had a knife at your throat. Your heart rate would probably increase, your muscles would tighten and your breathing would speed up. Many other changes would occur as well. Your body would automatically begin hormonal alterations and biochemical changes in the brain. Take a look at the following chart, which summarizes some of the ways your body is affected by the fight-or-flight response controlled by the sympathetic nervous system.

Stress and the Autonomic Nervous System

Body Part	Sympathetic	Parasympathetic
Eyes	pupils dilate	pupils constrict
Heart rate	increases	decreases
Blood vessels	constrict	dilate
Skeletal muscles	tighten	relax
Digestion	shuts down	works normally
Pancreas	inhibits insulin secretion	promotes insulin secretion
Sweat glands	increase secretion	secrete normally
Brain	secretes adrenaline	functions normally

The body's ability to do all of this automatically in order to protect itself is truly amazing. The pupils dilate to let more light in so that you can see more clearly if you are in danger. Digestion shuts down because it is not important in times of real emergency when the body's energy is needed elsewhere. The pancreas inhibits the secretion of insulin so you will have a higher blood sugar level to give you extra energy. Adrenaline is secreted to give you more strength than you would have normally.

Let's look at two changes the fight-or-flight response triggers in the nervous system: muscle tension and blood flow. All animals, including humans, have an unconscious instinct to tighten up the neck and shoulder muscles when they feel threatened. This occurs because animals instinctively try to protect the throat, which is where most animals are attacked. The neck and shoulder area is almost always the first place people experience muscle tension because of this programmed physiological response to a threat.

Many people, including those with migraines and high blood pressure, respond to stress by constricting their blood vessels. Animals, including human animals, tighten the muscles around the blood vessels so they will bleed less if they are attacked. The blood goes away from the extremities and towards the viscera, or primary organs, in the main part of the body. This is one more of the body's remarkable tricks for protecting itself in the presence of perceived danger.

Today, most of our stressors are psychological rather than physical. For example, we might be stuck in a traffic jam, have problems with our computer working properly or feel rushed to get everything done in too little time. Unfortunately, our bodies react to psychological stressors in the same way they react to physical dangers. This can be very damaging physiologically because we usually have no outlet for the hormones and tension that build up in the body from psychological stress. If it were a physical danger that threatened us, we would be able to release the adrenaline and tension from the body by running or fighting.

Having an over-aroused nervous system has become the norm in our fast-paced, competitive society where we live in a state of constant information overload. Modern society can keep people in a perpetual state of stress. Our wonderfully adaptive bodies begin to consider a high state of stress in our nervous systems as normal. This situation is difficult to avoid because even people who do not have many personal stressors still experience tension related to world and social conditions.

Unless people know how to release the stress that builds up in their body and mind, there will unquestionably be physical damage as a result. It can take the form of high blood pressure, ulcers, anxiety, insomnia, migraine headaches or numerous other disorders.

However, stress does not have to be physically, psychologically or emotionally damaging. It is not so much what happens in our lives that causes our nervous system stress as how we react to what happens in life. I remember reading once that a poll was taken to determine what events in life caused people the most stress. Speaking in public was ranked as the most stressful event, while dying was ranked at number four. Apparently, most people would rather die than speak in front of a group of people! However, there are those people who love to get up in front of others and give a talk. It doesn't make their heart beat faster or their palms sweat; their nervous system is not adversely affected in any way. This is because they are not reacting to the situation. In this training, you will learn how to respond to situations that life presents rather than reacting. As a result, you will not trigger your nervous system to shift to the sympathetic fight-or-flight response.

Eustress, Distress and Dis-ease

What few of us realize is that a good or positive event can bring as much stress to the body and mind as a bad or negative event. We all know that when someone close to us dies, we experience what we would call a bad stress or *distress*. But good stressors can affect the body in the same way. For example, perhaps you are getting married and are very excited and happy about it. This can still be a stress even though it is a good stress, or what we call *eustress*. The body's physiological response is the same to eustress as it is to distress.

Disease, or *dis-ease*, comes from being ill at ease in the body and/or mind. When we are not at ease with life we get out of balance.

We lose our homeostasis and our innate ability to fight off disease. This program is about bringing balance back into your life and your nervous system. It has far-reaching benefits beyond what you are probably imagining right now.

Biofeedback and Biofeedback Skills

Biofeedback is short for "biological feedback." It is a way to measure, control and balance your autonomic nervous system. In biofeedback we attach instruments to your body that measure such things as muscle tension, heart rate, blood flow through the arteries, sweat gland activity and respiration. Biofeedback is a way to see what is going on within your body by using instruments to amplify the subtle signals generated by the body. As you begin to recognize and understand these signals, you can learn to consciously control certain bodily functions that you don't usually control voluntarily.

Biofeedback skills are the tools and techniques people learn in order to control their signals, or readings, on the biofeedback instruments. You will be learning the same techniques in this book that I would teach a patient in my clinical biofeedback practice. This book will teach you the skills you need to know to control your ANS. It is not crucial to your success to have a biofeedback monitor in order to master the skills. However, some people find little home biofeedback units to be a good and inexpensive way to monitor their progress. If you would like to use a home unit, go to the website at the bottom of this page to find a selection of home biofeedback monitors.

Biofeedback skills are extremely effective for helping people to reduce or eliminate pain, headaches and stress in the body. We live in chaotic times; everyone's nervous system is under assault. This constant stress does take a toll on the physical body and affects the brain chemistry since the brain is a major part of the nervous system. Some estimate that more than 90 percent of doctor visits are from stress-related illnesses, so biofeedback, which helps bring balance and peace to the body and mind, could benefit many.

Symptoms and Causes of Stress

In the beginning of this lesson you answered many questions, which hopefully led you to think about some of the specific symptoms and possible triggers of your stress. In this section we will be addressing some of those questions that you answered. Now that you have a good understanding of how the autonomic nervous system works, it is time to look at the symptoms and causes of your stress in more depth. Familiarizing yourself with the symptoms will increase your awareness of what is occurring in your body so that you can make internal shifts to prevent the stress from turning into a serious physical or mental disorder.

Cold Hands and Feet

Did you answer "yes" when asked if you have a tendency towards cold hands and feet? People who have migraines or high blood pressure unconsciously constrict the blood vessels in their bodies. People with migraines constrict blood flow not only to their hands and feet, but also to the head. The brain and eyes need 80 percent of the body's blood and oxygen to function properly, so eventually the arteries need to open. When the arteries re-open to normal capacity after having been restricted, a migraine headache can be the result. This is caused by overcompensation during which the blood can go throbbing to the brain and eyes.

You may not experience cold hands and feet if you are taking medication that is a vasodilator. A vasodilator will keep the arteries open to prevent high blood pressure or a migraine. In the case of migraine, a vasoconstrictor, which tightens the arteries to slow down the flow of blood to the head, is often prescribed. Both are used for the treatment of migraines. Typically, people with migraines who are not on medications report cold hands and feet due to blood flow constriction. Even if you do not have either of these vascular symptoms, it will be helpful to your entire nervous system to learn how to consciously warm your hands and feet.

Medications that are vasodilators or vasoconstrictors can be a good temporary solution while you learn how to control your circulation. The sooner you take control of your blood flow the easier it will be. It can be more difficult to balance the nervous system if you have been on these medications for years or decades. But, keep going with the program and know that I have seen hundreds of people master their nervous systems after being on medications for decades.

Shoulder or Neck Pain or Stiffness

Do you have pain or stiffness in your shoulders or neck? Most readers probably answered "yes" to this question. If you answered "no," you may not be aware of what "normal" muscle tension is in your neck and shoulders. With biofeedback, we can measure the muscle tension in this area. Each muscle has a "normal" level of tension measured in microvolts.

If we don't feel pain or soreness in a muscle, we tend to think we have a normal level of tension. Since humans are such good adapters what we consider to be "normal" tension is usually very high. We adapt to stress and tension and then that becomes our normal. If you have headaches, or work on a computer all day, you almost certainly have a high level of tension in the neck and shoulder area. I recommend that everyone do the lessons on the neck and shoulders because most people have excess tension here. Remember, in the fight or flight response this is the first place tension usually goes.

Jaw Tension

Do you clench or grind your teeth during the day or night? Not everyone holds stress in the jaw area. This is one lesson you could potentially skip if you are absolutely certain you have no excess tension in the jaw area. However, as discussed above, we frequently simply adapt to excess muscle tension and are therefore often unaware that we are experiencing it. If you aren't sure whether or not you have tension in the jaw area, please do this lesson. If you have a guard that you wear in your mouth at night, it is important to understand that this guard, while it will protect your teeth, will not address the problem of clenching or tension in the jaw. It does not get to the root cause of the problem. Jaw tension can radiate into the temple and into other muscle groups in the head and cause muscle tension headaches. Jaw tension, clenching or grinding can also ruin your teeth and result in expensive dental treatment that is often preventable.

Eyestrain

Do you ever experience eyestrain? Most people do. The eyes can get strained in many ways, from lighting that is not full spectrum, looking at a computer for too long, reading, and even from emotional stress. However, because not all people experience eyestrain, this is another lesson that you could possibly skip. But, if you wear glasses or your eyesight is not perfect, even if you don't think you experience eyestrain, I recommend that you do this lesson. You might find your eyesight improving in addition to eliminating tension in the muscles surrounding the eyes. The tension in these muscles can be a contributing factor to your muscle tension headaches.

Caffeine and Cigarettes

Do you drink coffee; ingest any other caffeine or smoke cigarettes? If you answered "yes" to any part of this question, you might want to make some lifestyle changes to help keep your body in the parasympathetic nervous system. Caffeine and nicotine both stimulate the sympathetic nervous system. They cause the skeletal muscles to tense and the arteries to constrict. You can easily start weaning yourself from coffee by mixing caffeinated coffee with decaffeinated coffee. Other sources of caffeine include tea, chocolate, diet pills and over-the-counter medications such as acetaminophen with added caffeine. If you suffer from migraine headaches cutting out caffeine is critical.

If you smoke cigarettes, it is now time to cut back and eventually stop smoking entirely. Consult with your doctor on the best way for you to do this. There are many options to help with this, including classes, hypnotherapy and patches to name a few. I will not be mentioning caffeine or nicotine again. Just know that both of these substances are sympathetic nervous system stimulators.

Making Your Stress Chart

For the greatest benefit you will want to create a concise chart to track your symptoms of stress, their intensity level, triggers, medications and routine for staying on track. I find the best way to chart is

Stress Chart

Name _____ Month _____ Year _____

	1	2	3	4	5	6	7	8	9	10	11	12	13	14	15	16	17	18	19	20	21	22	23	24	25	26	27	28	29	30	31	
Morning																																1 - Mild
Afternoon																																2 - Moderate
Evening																																3 - Severe
Sleep																																4 - Incapacitating

	1	2	3	4	5	6	7	8	9	10	11	12	13	14	15	16	17	18	19	20	21	22	23	24	25	26	27	28	29	30	31	
Medication																																Tally
1 _____																																1 _____
2 _____																																2 _____
3 _____																																3 _____
4 _____																																4 _____
5 _____																																5 _____

	1	2	3	4	5	6	7	8	9	10	11	12	13	14	15	16	17	18	19	20	21	22	23	24	25	26	27	28	29	30	31	
Breathing Exercises																																X - on dates
Deep Relaxation																																X - on dates
Shoulder Exercises																																X - on dates
Neck Exercises																																X - on dates
Jaw Exercises																																X - on dates
Eye Exercises																																X - on dates
Triggers																																Triggers
Temp. Training																																X - on dates

FIGURE 2.1
Stress chart.

with a numbering system where you can have an entire month on one sheet. To have a separate sheet for every single day would be tedious, and it is not as easy to see the overall picture that way.

Make your stress chart sideways on an 8½ x 11-inch sheet of paper. This way you will be able to fit 31 days going across. Refer to figure 2.1 for creating your chart. You might be able to enlarge the chart on the following page so that it is usable without recreating it. Symptoms of stress would include, but not be limited to, the following: anxiety, insomnia, panic attacks, ulcers, essential hypertension, headaches, pain, irritable bowel syndrome, bruxism or other TMJ disorders. You might want to track symptoms that are exacerbated by stress such as fibromyalgia, chronic pain, or depression. Modify your chart so that it works for you and includes the symptoms you are working to improve.

How to Use Your Stress Chart

Your stress chart is an important record for several reasons. First, you will want to have an accurate record of your improvement. Sometimes it is hard to remember just how much improvement you have made. Second, this chart will be important for your doctor to see when you go for visits. Third, it is helpful to see if there are any triggers that increase your stress. Finally, your stress chart will make it easy to see whether or not you are staying on track with the exercises and activities you will be doing so that you're sure not to forget any of them.

Once a day, preferably right before bedtime, record on your chart. First, record your symptoms and their intensity level. This is done with a numbering system: 1=mild, 2=moderate, 3=severe and 4=incapacitating. If you did not have any symptoms, you can leave the box blank or put in a dash. You will see that there is a breakdown according to the time of day.

Next, record any medications you took during the day that may be relevant to your symptoms. This should include both over-the-counter and prescription drugs. In the appropriate box write down the number of pills you had during the day. For example, if you had two acetaminophen tablets during the day, put "2" in the box. At the end of each month you will be able to easily tally how many of each medication you took.

Next, make a numbered list of triggers at the bottom of the chart. I like people to make their own trigger list. Think about some things that might trigger your symptoms. When you have symptoms that are moderate to incapacitating in intensity, think about what might have been the trigger. Put the number(s) that correlates to that trigger in the appropriate box. Add to your trigger list as you become aware of, or remember, more triggers. This way, you can identify and then take care to avoid triggers as much as possible.

Finally, chart your routine for staying on track. This will simply require a check next to each skill you practiced on a particular day. Notice the chart in figure 2.1. You will see a column for the relaxation tape, breathing exercises, shoulder exercises and so on. As you move through this program you will have more and more skills to practice and probably will not get to all of them every day. The chart will help you to notice the exercises you haven't done in a few days, so you can rotate appropriately.

This system for having an entire month on one sheet is something you will appreciate once you start doing it. My clients have found that it is very easy and efficient. Over the years, I have often seen people tracking their symptoms in their day planner or on separate sheets each day. This new system makes it much easier to get an immediate overview of your improvement. Your doctor will also appreciate being able to easily read this chart. If you would like to make more notes, simply put them on the back of the sheet. For example, sometimes people like to note that they went on vacation, worked an excessive amount of time or anything else that might be relevant.

Save your monthly charts in a folder so you can see your progress as you move through this program. Obviously, you should see the number and intensity of symptoms declining and the intake of relevant medications being reduced as you master the skills you are learning. Sometimes it is easy to forget the progress that has been made, especially when in the midst of a relapse. That's why it is extremely helpful to have the progress documented in writing.

Practice

Make your stress chart format and copies of it before proceeding to the next chapter. Start charting immediately. Get in the habit of charting every single day.

Now that you are fully committed to the program, understand the physiological changes that are necessary and have started your stress chart, it is time to begin learning some new skills.

3

Calm the Body/
Still the Mind

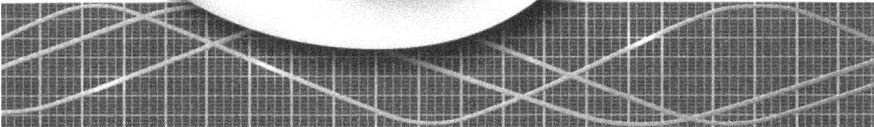

Body Awareness and the Body-Mind Connection

Most people are more aware of things outside of themselves than they are of their own bodies. Right now, for example, you might be more aware of what time it is or what you are going to eat at your next meal than you are of your body. Body awareness is the first step in recognizing the tension you carry in your nervous system. The next step is learning how to effectively release that tension.

In this section of the book you will become more aware of your body as a whole. The body is in large part a reflection of all that is going on in your mind and emotions. Learning how to calm the body and still the mind is a critical step to eliminating your symptoms of stress. You will be learning and practicing three important skills to help you calm the body and still the mind: proper breathing, deep relaxation and intentional imagining, or the use of imagery.

Typically, the body registers stress before the conscious mind does. If you listen to your body, you will become well aware of when your nervous system is shifting into an aroused state. Muscle tension, constricted breathing and cold hands and feet are just a few examples of your body letting you know that you are experiencing stress.

The mind and body are so intimately connected that they cannot be separated if one is to effectively treat any physical disorder. A term I like to use is the body-mind. When you create deep relaxation in the body, it is not possible to experience psychological stress. Likewise, when you still the mind, the body begins to relax. Deep relaxation of the body and mind is incompatible with anxiety, tension and many physical disorders.

The next three lessons will help you to create what I like to call a "new normal" level of tension in your body. These general skills will help you begin regulating your breathing and heart rate, reduce muscle tension and increase blood flow or circulation.

Breathing Your
Way to Relaxation

Breathing Correctly to Calm the Body-Mind

The easiest and best way to create a shift in your autonomic nervous system is with proper breathing. Remember, shifting your ANS into homeostasis will cause your arteries to dilate and your muscles to relax, two critical components in improving your health. The reason I like to start with breathing is that it is extremely effective and can be practiced anytime and anywhere. You can use it if you are stressed while stuck in traffic, waiting in a line, or at a meeting. Proper breathing will calm the body and help relax the mind.

Before reading this chapter, try this exercise: place one hand on your chest and one hand on your belly below the navel, and notice how you are breathing without changing your breath in any way. What happens when you inhale? Does your chest expand or does it contract? Is there any movement in the belly when you inhale? If there is, does the belly expand or contract?

Now, using a clock with a second hand, count the number of breaths you breathe in the next fifteen seconds. Multiply that by four to get your number of breaths per minute. Write this number down to remember it. While counting breaths, did you breathe in and out of your nose or did you use your mouth to breathe? Did your breathing feel tight or constricted in any way? Were the breaths regular or irregular in their rhythm? Pay attention to every detail of your breathing.

Diaphragmatic Breathing vs. Thoracic Breathing

As I mentioned in the first chapter, everything we do is a habit. Your way of breathing is a very old habit that you developed as a young child. This early childhood pattern usually stays with people for a lifetime unless they consciously work on learning to breathe correctly.

Have you ever watched infants breathe? If you have, you may have noticed that they breathe full, deep, diaphragmatic breaths. Their bellies rise as they inhale and drop down as they exhale. Unfortunately, in our modern society, they pick up on the stress around them at a very young age and soon develop poor breathing patterns.

Thoracic breathers primarily breathe in their chests. If you noticed that you had little or no movement in your belly while breathing, you are a thoracic breather. At least 40 percent of the people I have worked with in my practice are thoracic, or chest, breathers when they first come to me. Thoracic breathing creates anxiety, stress and muscle tension by throwing the whole ANS into the sympathetic realm. In other words, just by breathing improperly we can shift the whole nervous system into the fight-or-flight response. On the other hand, simply by breathing correctly we can shift the nervous system into the parasympathetic or relaxed mode.

Most people use a very small percentage of their lung capacity with each breath. The lung's capacity is approximately 6,000 cubic centimeters per breath but the average person uses only 500 cubic centimeters per breath, or one twelfth of his or her total lung capacity. It is important to start taking in more air per breath by filling the lungs as completely as possible. This will slow down the number of breaths per minute.

How many breaths per minute (BPM) were you breathing when you did the previous exercise? The average person breathes approximately 16 breaths per minute. I have seen people breathing as much as 32 to 34 BPM. Breathing this fast is almost like panting, and it is extremely damaging to both the body and the mental-emotional state. The ideal number of breaths per minute is six. This is what you will be striving to achieve. There is no advantage to getting below six breaths per minute.

You might think that six BPM sounds terribly slow. However, if you stop to think about it, that is only a five-second inhalation followed by a five-second exhalation, or ten seconds per breath. I have rarely had a patient that could not achieve this goal. I have seen some people get down to two breaths per minute. I would not suggest this as a normal breathing pattern, however. There is some debate as to whether it is healthy to slow down breathing that much.

I had one patient who was breathing 32 BPM at the beginning of a session. She was in her forties and had asthma, although that was not what she was seeing me for. Her eyes grew wide when I told her that the ideal number of breaths per minute was six, and she exclaimed, "I'll never be able to do that!" I told her that even if she got down to 12 BPM, that would be a huge improvement and an enormous help with her high blood pressure. By the end of the

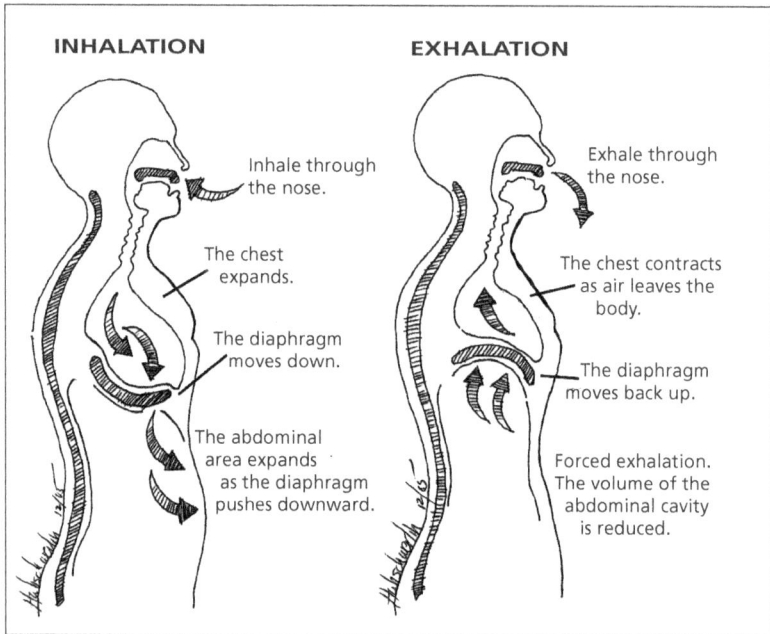

FIGURE 3.1—Proper inhalation and exhalation to calm the nervous system.

same session, to her amazement, she was down to 5 BPM. She was breathing smooth, even, deep breaths.

Several months later, she told me that this one lesson gave her more control over her asthma than anything in her entire life, including medications. She is a wonderful example of the incredible power of proper breathing!

The only muscles used when breathing correctly are the diaphragm and the intercostal muscles. The diaphragm is a very large muscle. It is about an inch thick and it separates the chest cavity from the abdominal cavity. As you inhale, your lungs fill with air and expand. This expansion causes the diaphragm to be pushed down resulting in expansion in the abdominal area. As you exhale, the diaphragm moves up, and there should then be contraction in the abdominal area and the chest as the air leaves the body (see figure 3.1). This up-and-down movement of the diaphragmatic muscle is very calming and relaxing. This natural process is also a wonderful internal massage for all the organs in this part of your body. It helps to bring blood and oxygen to these organs and that in turn improves their health and functioning.

The diaphragm should account for approximately 80 percent of the movement in your body as you breathe. If you have been a thoracic breather, and therefore have not been using the diaphragm very much, it may initially get tired as you begin to use it more. This muscle, like any other muscle that hasn't been used, can get out of shape. In this case, do not attempt diaphragmatic breathing 24 hours a day at first. You will need to build up to this slowly. Your diaphragm will grow stronger and more flexible with use.

The other muscle group that is used when you are breathing correctly is the intercostal muscles. This muscle group surrounds the ribcage and lifts it up and out as you inhale. These muscles should account for the other 20 percent of movement in your body as you breathe correctly.

It is crucial that you do *not* use your neck and shoulder muscles as you breathe. People often use these muscles while breathing, but this is the last place in your body you need more muscle tension! All the movement as you breathe should be in the front of your body, completely supported by the diaphragm and the intercostal muscles.

As you begin to deeply breathe, you will need to make a very conscious effort to be sure you are not tensing in the neck, shoulders or upper back. Initially, it will help to practice diaphragmatic breathing while lying down. This makes it easier to keep the neck and shoulder muscles relaxed while learning.

Breathe in and out through your nose, not your mouth. The body was designed for you to breathe this way, and there is a wonderful system in the nasal passages to filter out airborne bacteria. This system does not exist in the throat, making it more likely for you to catch colds, flus and other diseases that are airborne if you breathe through your mouth.

Try this simple exercise now so that you will know how it feels to breathe using the diaphragm. Sit in a chair, clasp your hands behind your neck, and bring the elbows apart. Take a deep breath and notice how you are breathing now. This simple movement will cause you to breathe diaphragmatically, and you will feel the difference immediately.

Benefits of Diaphragmatic Breathing

Let's first look at the benefits of diaphragmatic breathing in relationship to stress. Diaphragmatic breathing is a very effective way to dilate the arteries and increase your circulation. Your health and well-being will improve when you come to a place where your arteries are dilated and you can maintain that dilation. You may experience warming in your hands and feet when you begin to open your arteries.

Breathing properly will cause a shift in your entire ANS. Remember, the nervous system controls everything in your body, from your cardiovascular system to your digestive system. The health of your entire body can improve with proper breathing. Breathing exercises have been proven to be effective in reducing muscle tension, in addition to dilating the arteries.

Every cell in the body needs oxygen to be healthy and strong. With healthy cells you will create healthy tissues and organs. When we breathe properly, the toxins are carried out of each cell and eliminated as the carbon dioxide passes from the body. But when we are not breathing correctly, the toxins cannot be fully released from the body. These toxins, when held in the body, can lead to anxiety, depression and fatigue.

It is especially good to know that when you begin breathing correctly, you will dramatically improve the health of your heart. With each deep and full inhalation your heart rate will increase, and with each complete exhalation your heart rate will decrease. This is called heart rate variability. For example, as you inhale your heart rate might go up to 90 beats per minute, and as you exhale your heart rate might drop down to 50 **BPM**. This variability is a very good thing. It builds a strong and healthy heart.

The heartbeat directly follows the breathing. When I connect people to my biofeedback instruments and they have short, shallow breathing, I see absolutely no variability in their heart rate. But when they start breathing diaphragmatically, we immediately start to see the variability. There should be at least a 20-point variation in the heart rate between the inhalation and exhalation. For example, if your heart rate went up to 80 on the inhalation and dropped to 60 on the exhalation, you would have a 20-point spread. You do not actually have to see this on instruments. Just know that if you are breathing properly, you will have good heart rate variability.

Proper breathing habits are essential not only for your physical health but also for your psychological well-being. It is hard to maintain tension, stress, anger or anxiety while you are breathing properly. Studies show that depression, irritability and panic attacks are also reduced with diaphragmatic breathing. Proper breathing is an antidote to stress. It can bring a feeling of calm and relaxation when it is done purposefully. It can also make each stressful situation that you face many times easier to cope with.

Diaphragmatic Breathing Exercise

1. As you prepare to practice, be sure you are wearing loose, comfortable clothes. Find a quiet and relaxing place. Make sure the phone is turned off and you will not have any distractions. Now, lie down on your back on the floor or on a bed. Bend your legs at the knees. You might want to put a couple of pillows under the knees if that makes you more comfortable.

2. Place one hand on your belly below the navel and your other hand on the area just below the rib cage and above the navel (called *solar plexus*).

3. Close your eyes and become aware of how you are breathing.

4. Start breathing more consciously. Remember, you want to take in more air per breath and slow down the breaths per minute. As you inhale, focus on the chest, solar plexus and belly rising. Feel

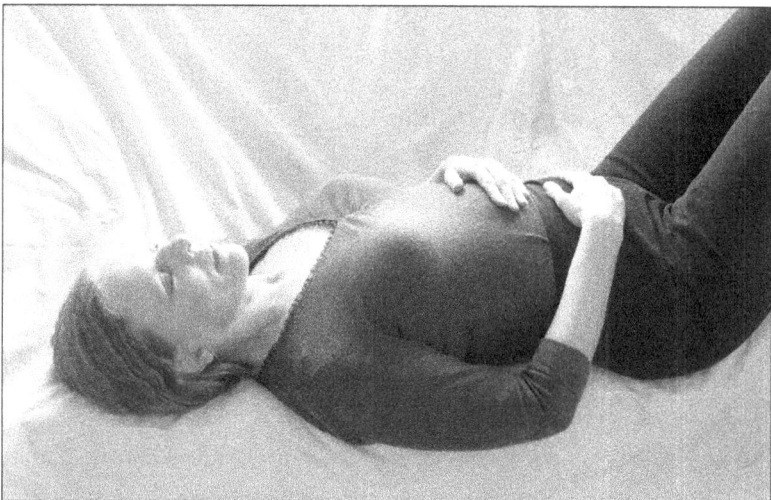

FIGURE 3.2
Inhalation with hands on solar plexus and belly.

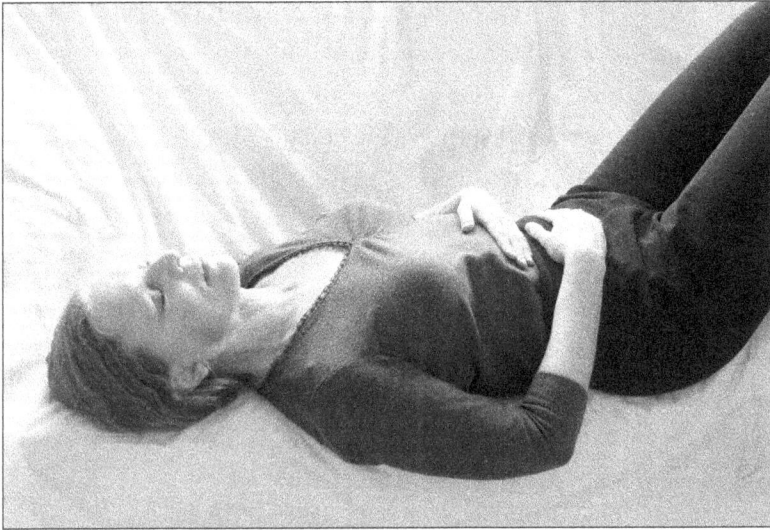

FIGURE 3.3
Practicing proper exhalation.

and imagine the air completely filling your lungs with the inhalation (fig. 3.2). With the exhalation, feel the chest, solar plexus and belly drop down as the air leaves the body. Be aware of the warm air leaving your body (fig. 3.3).

5. Continue practicing this slow, deep diaphragmatic breathing for ten minutes.

6. As you are breathing, notice which muscles are working. Are your neck and shoulder muscles totally relaxed?

While it is generally easiest to begin mastering this breathing technique while lying down, eventually you should be breathing this way while sitting, standing, walking and moving through your life. Ultimately, diaphragmatic breathing will become almost automatic, and this will be your new normal.

Still, you may have to consciously think about your breathing for some time before it becomes automatic. Remember, you may have had your current breathing pattern for decades. This new pattern may feel awkward at first, but with practice it will become second nature. Eventually, you will find that it creates a feeling of calm and stillness in both your body and mind.

Our society has taught us that we should have flat bellies. I say let your belly go! It is the only way you will be able to breathe dia-phragmatically. Women, especially, suck their bellies in and hold them in, preventing themselves from breathing fully. In recent years, many men feel this same social pressure. If you were taught to suck your belly in or decided to do so after being inundated with images of rail-thin models, know that this unhealthy idea is based on noth-ing more than current societal conditioning and serves neither your appearance nor your well-being. Learn to relax your belly. On the exhalation it is fine to tighten the abdominal muscles; this is, in fact, great exercise for those muscles. However, with the inhalation, you need to let those muscles relax.

Occasionally, people feel lightheaded when they begin breath-ing diaphragmatically. This is because they are slightly changing the carbon dioxide and oxygen levels in the blood. If this happens to you, stop the deep breathing and go back to your old pattern until the lightheadedness subsides. This just means you will need to take it a bit slower until your body adjusts. For example, instead of practic-ing for 10 minutes at a time, try five minutes. If that is still too much, start with three minutes at a time. You will probably find your body adjusting rather quickly and you will then be able to increase your time gradually.

It is especially important to focus on slow, regular, deep breath-ing any time you feel tension and want to bring peace and calmness to yourself. Also, if you have a problem sleeping, lie on your back with your hands on your chest and belly and focus on this breathing technique. You will be amazed how quickly you will calm yourself and fall asleep.

Practice

1. Practice the diaphragmatic exercise explained in this lesson ten minutes every day. Set aside time when you can focus totally on your breathing. Create a time and a space that is exclusively for your practice, and follow the instructions outlined above.

   People often ask me what time of day is best to practice. Any time of day is fine, so do what works best for you. Be consistent so you begin to create a new habit of breathing correctly. I suggest you find a routine time. It might be at lunchtime before eating or right before dinner.

2. In order to successfully integrate this breathing technique into your life, you need to be reminded often throughout the day. I give patients what I call "cue dots," which serve as a cue to remind people of their breathing. Find some color-coded labels or round color dots with sticky backs. Take about seven of these dots and put them in places where you will see them often—perhaps on your day planner, refrigerator, steering wheel or rear view mirror of your car, bathroom mirror, telephone at work, etc. Every time you see one of these dots, take a full, deep, diaphragmatic breath and hold it for a moment, if it is comfortable for you to do so. Next exhale slowly and completely. If holding after the inhalation is not comfortable, go straight into the exhalation. Only one deep breath is needed every time you see a dot; you will see the dots often throughout the day!

You will be using these dots as cues to remind you to practice new skills throughout this training. If they start to blend into the woodwork after a few weeks and you are not responding to them, then it is time to change the color. The dots will be significant in helping all your new habits to become more automatic. After all, you are creating a new normal in your autonomic nervous system, so you will need to be reminded often in the beginning.

Once again, remember that everything you do is a habit. In order to create this new normal in your ANS, you must replace your old breathing habit with your new breathing habit. To establish your new breathing pattern, it is important that you not move onto the next lesson until you have achieved some level of mastery with breathing properly.

Deep Relaxation
of the Body-Mind

Introduction to Self-Regulation

In biofeedback we teach what is called "self-regulation" of the autonomic nervous system. This simply means that you learn how to consciously regulate such things as muscle tension, heart rate and blood flow that are normally controlled by the ANS. One very effective way to learn self-regulation is with a technique called *autogenics*.

The goal of autogenics training is to teach you how to maintain your physical, mental and emotional processes at a normal level of tension no matter what is happening around you. These processes can all get out of balance due to stress. When you encounter an emotionally or physically stressful event, your body chemistry can become imbalanced, which can lead to numerous changes in the body-mind. Autogenics is very effective in training you how to bring your body-mind back to homeostasis, or a state of equilibrium.

Autogenics training was developed by Johannes Shultz, a Berlin psychiatrist, who found that we can create a state very much like a hypnotic trance by repeating mental messages of heaviness and warmth to the body. Shultz created this system in the 1930's. It has profound healing effects on the body-mind, which can be measured. The effects can be measured and proven by attaching biofeedback instruments. However, even without instruments you can be aware of how you feel before and after an autogenics exercise.

The script that follows integrates autogenics with my work. I have included body scanning and a relaxation of the mind in the script. In my experience, this makes the autogenics even more effective.

There are numerous benefits to mastering this body-mind re-laxation exercise. This deep relaxation exercise will help you begin to learn how to dilate your arteries, relax muscle tension, calm your heartbeat and remember to regulate and open your breathing. Addi-tionally, deep relaxation training such as this will help you to reduce irritability, fatigue and general anxiety. You can use it to help calm your reaction to pain and to increase your resistance to stress. It is also quite useful if you have a difficult time sleeping.

Recording Your Deep Relaxation Script

It is very difficult to focus on deep relaxation without having a tape or CD to follow. Without it, your mind will probably start to wander. Even with a recording, you might find your mind wander-ing. If your mind does wander, gently bring yourself back to the exercise. Work on focusing 100 percent of your attention to the ex-ercise as you practice.

Read the script slowly and clearly as you record. You might want to have some soothing, relaxing background music as you record, but this is a matter of personal taste. Make sure there will be no interruptions as you record the script.

Frequently people tell me they do not like to hear the sound of their own voice. If that is the case for you, have someone else record the script for you or order the deep relaxation CD, Calming the Body/Stilling the Mind, from the website listed at the bottom of this page. There is a free, 12-minute CD download on the homepage. However, first start with the full-length relaxation CD, which you can order from the store on the site. Use the full-length CD for at least two months. After some practice, you will be able to achieve the same results in a shorter period of time. When your ANS is under control and more balanced, you can choose to work with the shorter version if you prefer.

The Deep Relaxation Script

What you are about to experience is an exercise in deep relaxation of both the body and the mind. Make sure that you will not be interrupted for the next 25 minutes. Lie on a recliner or bed in a completely comfortable position, and make sure you will be warm. Uncross your legs and let your feet drop out to the sides as the legs begin to relax. Check to see that your arms are relaxed, loose and limp, and turn the palms upwards if that is comfortable.

Now take a deep, full inhalation, relaxing your belly as you inhale. Pause for a moment with the inhalation and then exhale, breathing out all the warm air. Take another deep, full breath and imagine this time, as you exhale, that you are breathing away any tension or anxiety you are holding in your body or mind. Continue this pattern of deep, rhythmic breathing throughout the exercise.

Begin by letting your mind relax. Be aware of the thoughts in your mind, but imagine that you are watching them from a distance…almost as if each thought were a white puffy cloud against the clear blue sky. You are fully aware of your thoughts, but you don't let any of them disturb your sense of inner peace. Don't cling to any of the thoughts…just watch them as they float on by. They don't control you or your life; you know that you are the master of your thoughts, your mind. The thoughts, just like the clouds, sometimes appear from nowhere…and sometimes they disappear…just like the clouds. You just watch. Some of the clouds may seem very large and others much smaller. You remain undisturbed…a witness to the thoughts you see. Now imagine the clouds…the thoughts…beginning to disappear…evaporating into space…as your mind becomes more calm and clear…as it peacefully rests in quiet serenity. Finally all you see is the clear blue sky, just like the clarity of your consciousness.

As your mind becomes more calm and clear, it will be easier to focus on relaxing the various parts of your body.

Now bring your awareness to your legs and feet. Be aware of how your legs and feet feel. Scan them, noticing the heels of your feet, the balls of your feet, the arches, the tops of your feet and the toes. Scan up through the ankles, lower legs, knees and thighs. Let all the muscles here relax, going loose and limp, and repeat to yourself, "My legs are heavy and relaxed. My legs are heavy and relaxed. My legs are heavy and relaxed." Feel the heaviness in your legs. Feel your legs sinking into the surface you are lying upon as they relax totally.

Now shift your awareness to your shoulders. Let your shoulders drop. Scan through the upper arms, elbows, lower arms, wrists, hands, the top of the hands, the back of the hands, and the fingers—right down to the tip of every finger. Let all the muscles in your arms and hands relax completely, and say to yourself, "My arms and hands are heavy. My arms and hands are heavy. My arms and hands are heavy." Be aware of the heaviness as you go deeper and deeper into relaxation. Allow the surface you are laying on to support the weight of your arms.

Now bring your awareness to your neck and shoulder area. Consciously relax the muscles here. Feel your head just sinking into whatever surface you are lying on as you relax these muscles. Say to yourself, "My neck and shoulders are heavy. My neck and shoulders are heavy. My neck and shoulders are heavy." Feel the heaviness here.

Now bring your awareness back to your legs and feet. Imagine a feeling of warmth all the way down to your feet and your toes as you dilate the arteries here. Say to yourself, "My legs and feet are warm. My legs and feet are warm. My legs and feet are warm." Feel the warmth and the heaviness in your legs and in your feet.

Return your awareness to your shoulders, arms and hands. Imagine the feeling of warmth here increasing as you relax the arteries in this part of your body. Imagine the blood flow and circulation increasing all the way down to your fingertips. Feel the warmth and say to yourself, "My arms and hands are warm. My arms and hands are warm. My arms and hands are warm." Feel the warmth and the heaviness in your arms and in your hands.

Bring your awareness back to your neck and shoulders. Imagine the muscles here being bathed in blood and oxygen. Feel the warmth as you increase the circulation here and say to yourself, "My neck and shoulders are warm. My neck and shoulders are warm. My neck and shoulders are warm." Feel the warmth and the heaviness in your neck and shoulders.

Now move your awareness to your breathing. Feel the air completely filling your lungs with the inhalation, and with the exhalation feel the warm air leaving your body. Breathe out any tension with each exhalation and breathe in relaxation and peace with every inhalation. Imagine the relaxation and peace going to each and every cell. Say to yourself, "My breathing is calm and regular. My breathing is calm and regular. My breathing is calm and regular." With each full and deep breath, you nourish all the cells in your body, and you bring your body back to a place of total well-being.

Now bring your attention to your heart as you begin to calm and regulate your heartbeat. Say to yourself, "My heartbeat is calm and regular. My heartbeat is calm and regular. My heartbeat is calm and regular."

Move your awareness now to your abdominal area. Relax all the muscles here and imagine all the internal organs relaxing so they can function more perfectly. Take a deep abdominal breath as you expand the belly area. Pause for a moment with the inhalation and then exhale fully and completely. Take another deep, full breath, and as you exhale say to yourself, "My abdomen is calm and relaxed. My abdomen is calm and relaxed. My abdomen is calm and relaxed."

Bring your awareness to your forehead now as you let the muscles here begin to relax. Relax the muscles on the sides of your head, the top of your head, and the back of your head. Relax the temples. Relax the muscles that surround the eyes and relax the eyes themselves. Let all the muscles in the head and face become free of any tension. Then imagine any excess blood in the head drifting away from the head and going towards the hands and the feet as you experience a feeling of coolness in your head and warmth in your hands and feet—as you redirect the blood flow in your body. Now say to yourself, "My forehead is cool and calm. My forehead is cool and calm. My forehead is cool and calm."

Now bring your attention to your whole body–being aware of each and every place from your feet to the top of your head to the tips of your fingers–giving each place in your body equal and simultaneous attention. Notice how good it feels to be completely relaxed and at peace with yourself. Know that you can recreate this feeling of relaxation any time you wish with some practice. Wherever you are, you have the power to bring your body to this place of relaxation and peace. If you are about to go to sleep now, say to yourself, "I sleep peacefully all through the night. I sleep peacefully all through the night. I sleep peacefully all through the night."

If you are ready to get up and continue on with your day, say to yourself, "I am refreshed and completely alert. I am refreshed and completely alert. I am refreshed and completely alert." Stretch your arms and your legs. Take a deep breath. Open your eyes when you are ready. Enjoy the feeling of being relaxed and energized at the same time.

Preparing to Practice Deep Relaxation

You will now use the recorded script to practice deep relaxation. Prepare for this exercise in the same way you prepared for the deep breathing practice: wear loose, comfortable clothing and be sure you will be warm and comfortable. Lie on a bed with a couple of pillows under your knees (fig. 4.1) or on a recliner that supports your head. Turn the telephone ringer off and make sure you will be free of all distractions.

You will receive the greatest benefits if you practice with all your attention focused upon the exercise. Eliminate external and internal distractions as much as possible. You might imagine that you are setting any worries, concerns or busyness in the mind outside the door of the room in which you are practicing. Know that these problems will be there when you come out if you chose to pick them up. It's okay

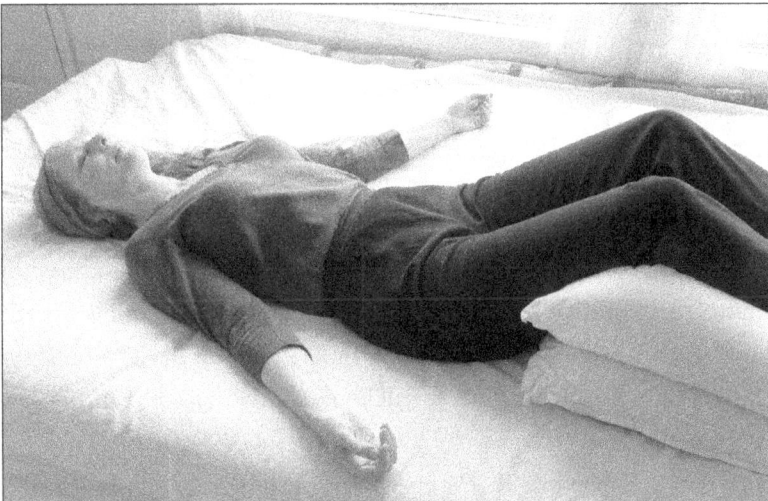

FIGURE 4.1
Preparing for deep relaxation.

to set all that aside for a little while. Those concerns may seem much smaller when you finish the exercise and are ready to leave the room.

It is best to practice this exercise while fully awake and alert. You need to learn how to be awake and relaxed rather than having to be asleep to be relaxed. Never practice this exercise, or any imagery or deep relaxation exercise, while driving a motor vehicle. Do your best to stay awake during the entire exercise. One trick I use successfully with my patients is to have them hold the lower part of one arm up in the air while resting the elbow on the chair and allowing the hand to relax loose and limp. If they start to fall asleep, the arm will begin to fall and will bring them back to waking consciousness. You can use this effective trick as well.

Anchoring

Anchoring is a technique that many people find helpful in training their ANS. It is a way for the body to remember to return to a normal level of tension even when there is an external stressor present. The simple act of bringing the thumb and middle finger together while you are practicing your deep relaxation exercise can be your anchor. The nervous system will associate this gesture with a calm and relaxed state of body and mind. Then, when you find your body reacting to an external stressor, you can simply bring the thumb and middle finger together while taking a deep slow breath, and your nervous system will remember to come back to homeostasis. When this happens, you will know that you have your nervous system effectively trained.

Whether you use anchoring or not during deep relaxation is an individual choice. Many of my patients find it helpful while others do not like the feeling of tension in their hand needed to hold this position. Find what works best for you. The anchor does not have to be the thumb and middle finger together. Perhaps resting your hand on your hipbone is the best anchor for you.

Charting Your Success

For many people, *feeling* the difference in their body and mind after practicing deep relaxation is enough to remind them of their progress. Some people prefer to record their progress. Recording will make you more aware of the drop in general tension that comes with continued practice. If you choose to record, simply keep a little notebook in the room where you will practice. Before the session, rank your level of general tension in the body and mind on a scale of one to ten, with one being totally relaxed/having no tension and ten being extremely tense/as tense as you can imagine being.

Note the date and rank your tension, writing it down before you start. Then practice your deep relaxation exercise. Before you get up at the end of the exercise, bring your awareness to your body and mind and rank your level of relaxation again. Write that number down. If you have any comments you would like to make a note of, write them down as well.

If you have the *Stress Mess Workbook*, you can find this chart already prepared for you. Each chart includes space for recording one week of practice, and you can make photocopies of the blank chart.

Practice

1. Practice the deep relaxation exercise with the tape at least once a day. This will shift your ANS into a more balanced place, helping you to reduce your stress-induced symptoms. As with

the breathing exercise, it is best to pick a consistent time each day to do this. It would be fine to combine your ten minutes of deep breathing with this exercise. People today have very busy lives, yet it is still important to continue with the deep breathing as a practice. If time is an issue, simply do them together.

If you do not get a chance to practice the deep relaxation exercise during the day and you need to practice right before bed, there is a good chance you will fall asleep during the exercise. Occasionally, this is fine. I believe it is more beneficial to practice while drifting off to sleep than to skip a day. But, of course, it is better to practice most of the time when you can be fully awake for the entire exercise. What is most important, however, is that you stay in the habit of daily practice. You may only consciously hear a few minutes of the tape sometimes, but your subconscious mind will hear all of the messages on the tape.

2. Are you staying on track with your stress chart, the cue dots, and your diaphragmatic breathing?

Imagery

Imagery and the Mind-Body Connection

For the past 300 years, Western medicine has operated as if the mind were separate from the body. You might be surprised to learn that no other medical system in the history of the world has made such a distinction. Even Western medicine before the seventeenth century did not separate the body and mind in healing. Western medicine today is finally beginning to acknowledge once again that everything a person thinks, believes and feels is experienced in the body. In fact, the mind and body are one inseparable system.

Interestingly, Western medicine does acknowledge that the physical can affect the mental. For example, when people are in chronic pain, they are often given anti-depressants and sleep medications because doctors understand that chronic pain can lead to depression and insomnia. Yet Western science has been reluctant to embrace the idea that the mind can alter the body. Since it is so obvious, and accepted, that the body can affect the mind, does it not stand to reason that we can affect the physical body with our thoughts and emotions?

Every thought and image that goes through the mind creates not only a chemical change in the brain, but also an electrical change in the nervous system. In other words, a biological change is triggered by every thought, belief and feeling. Every cell, tissue and organ is affected by the mind. If a healthcare provider ever tells you that some physical condition is "all in your mind," you can rest assured that there is a physical event going on as well. If it is in your mind, it is in your body as well–and vice versa.

The use of imagery is one of the most powerful methods to make shifts in the mind-body system. Now it is time for you to become the master of your mind and nervous system. As you know, the nervous system controls everything in the body. Intentional imagery can have a profound effect on your nervous system, which in turn will affect your overall well-being.

The Power of Imagery in Healing

The word *imagery* comes from the same root as *imagination*. We use our imaginations all the time whether we are consciously aware of it or not. Architects, for example, use imagination to visualize a building before making a drawing. Every building started as a creation of someone's imagination.

Today, people are learning to consciously control their imaginations for a variety of beneficial reasons. Olympic athletes, for example, imagine themselves over and over again performing their sport exactly as they want to create it in the physical plane. This has proven to be very effective in improving athletes' performance. Over the past few decades, the use of imagery has also become more acceptable in healing as there have been many scientific studies proving how effective it can be.

Usually when people hear the word *imagination*, they think of visual images. Yet, when we imagine we often include much more than the visual images. Imagery can also include the senses of taste, touch, smell and hearing.

The images in your mind can be either spontaneous or directed. *Spontaneous imagination* is produced by your subconscious mind. It arises of its own accord and includes all of your experiences, even those that you don't consciously remember. Spontaneous imagination is governed by your beliefs about yourself and life, which come from conditioned habits of thought. Most people are not very aware of the spontaneous images that constantly pass through their minds. Your dreams are one example of spontaneous images. Both night dreams and daydreams can be spontaneous.

Directed imagination, on the other hand, is the deliberate use of the power of your mind to create your own reality. Images are self-fulfilling prophecies. What you envision in life is what you get, whether that envisioning is conscious or unconscious. We can program what we want to create with images. Learning to use imagery as a tool for healing is an act of conscious and deliberate creating. You might think of it as creating a movie in your mind where you are the director. In this lesson, you will learn how you can consciously direct these inner movies for the benefit of your health and well-being.

Your Creative Mind

Tapping into your creative mind is essential in learning to successfully use imagery as a tool. Your creative mind is always working although you may not always be aware of it. For example, sometimes you just "know" something. It may not seem logical or based on science, but you know it to be the truth. You may at times hear an "inner voice" guiding you. These are just a couple of examples that you might relate to where you have tapped into the creative mind, which goes beyond logic.

The creative mind, the part of the mind we use when we imagine, is a right-brain experience. It bypasses the limitations of rational, analytical, linear thinking, tapping into the limitless source of personal power through intuition, creativity and imagination. Feeling and "knowing" are associated with the right side of the brain as well.

Left-brain thinking has been predominant in our Western society over the past several centuries. The left-brain can be a powerful tool when analyzing something, figuring out a problem or making decisions. Words govern the left hemisphere of the brain while images govern the right hemisphere of the brain. Unfortunately, the left-brain has been overused at the expense of the equally important right-brain. Learning how to tap into your creative mind will begin to unleash your real power, including the power to heal your own body.

Occasionally, people find it challenging to consciously control their mental images. Their minds simply wander aimlessly and control their lives. If you are a person who is controlled by your thoughts, you will achieve a true sense of freedom and empowerment when you begin to take control of your mental activity.

Sometimes people say they can't picture things in their mind because they think with words more than images. If you are one of these people, try recalling dreams or a pleasant experience, or visualize the face of someone you love. You will find that when you practice using images, you will be able to work with this language just as easily as the language of words. It is a skill that can be learned. For some people it flows very naturally while others need more practice.

It is important to remember that imagery is about more than seeing pictures. As was mentioned earlier, it can include all of your senses. You may become aware of a feeling impression, and that is also fine. You can relax into trusting that however you use your imagination is valid. Your favorite song may bring your sense of hearing into the forefront. If you are recalling a delicious meal, you may be more in touch with your sense of taste. While imagining walking through a rose garden, you are likely in touch with your sense of smell. When you imagine you are making love, you may be more in tune with your sense of touch. And, of course, you may be aware of several senses coming into play at the same time when using imagination.

Preparing for Imagery – Intention

The first step in preparing your mind for imagery is to be clear about your intention. Intention is what we wish to achieve. It is our desire. Intention is intimately connected with successful imaging. It directs both our attention and our action.

When we do intentional, or directed, imagery we begin by clarifying our intention. For example, you might intend to deeply relax all the muscles in your body during the imagery exercise. It could be that your intention is to calm and still the mind so you feel more at peace. My intention after a ski injury was to heal the primary ligament in the knee with imagery to avoid undergoing knee surgery.

With intention you become clear about what you want and tell yourself what you are going to accomplish. You are giving yourself an inner instruction. This directed will is essential to successfully using directed imagination.

Most people use their will to focus on external events or to create things they want from the material world. People shape their outer worlds with their will and intention. But sometimes will and intention alone are not enough because there are unconscious images sabotaging what the conscious mind says it wants to create. Regardless, I am sure you can think of many things you have created using your will and intention. You may be living in a house that you imagined or driving the car that you imagined. Your job or career is something you perhaps consciously imagined. I imagined writing a book on managing stress, and here it is! It was in my imagination long before it was in print.

We forget that we can turn that directed attention towards ourselves to make changes inwardly. We can use that power to take charge of the health in our bodies and minds. You will feel very exhilarated and empowered when you become the conscious master of your life by using your imagination and intention. Affecting your own healing can be one of the most rewarding experiences of your life. It can be much more empowering than turning your health over to another person.

Preparing for Imagery – Relaxation and Brain Waves

The human brain is the most powerful healing tool available to us. It is in a constant state of electrical activity in which it is emitting brain waves of varying frequency and amplitude. Our brains produce beta, alpha, theta and delta waves. When you are in your normal busy waking state of consciousness, your brain produces primarily beta waves. As you start to relax, the brain waves begin to shift into alpha. You undoubtedly experienced this shift in the previous lesson when you practiced the deep relaxation exercise. From this state you may become even more deeply relaxed, moving into theta brain waves. Finally, as the waves slow even more, the brain shifts into delta waves, which are associated with sleep.

It is important to relax your body-mind deeply so that you move into this slower brain-wave pattern. Your subconscious mind is much more receptive to healing and positive images, and to manifesting them into reality, when you are in a very relaxed state of mind. When your brain is producing alpha or theta waves, you will be far more effective in creating the changes you want in your body and in your life.

In order to make the shift from beta to alpha waves and to prepare yourself for effective imagery, you simply need to practice relaxation of the body and mind. Do a minimum of five to ten minutes of deep relaxation to prepare yourself to work with directed imagery. It is best to have a recorded relaxation tape directing you so that your mind does not wander. You can download a shortened (12-minute) version of *Calming the Body/Stilling the Mind* free from the website listed at the bottom of this page to deepen your relaxation before practicing imagery. You will find that the imagery script that follows starts with a short relaxation of the body and mind, which you will record on the tape before recording the directed imagery.

It can be especially powerful to practice your directed imagery at night just before sleeping or in the morning just after waking. At these times, your mind and body are usually already deeply relaxed and receptive. You are also probably in an alpha or theta brain-wave state where your imagery can be most powerful and effective. If you do this practice at night while lying in bed, try not to fall asleep. You can use the trick I mentioned in the previous chapter in which you bring the lower part of one arm up, balancing it on the elbow while relaxing the hand to stay awake.

Using intention and deep relaxation will allow your imagery to touch the deepest part of your being—your essence, your core—and allow you to achieve healing from a deeper place. From this place you will be able to manifest positive change far more effectively than by thinking, planning or trying to manipulate people and things. Remember, you are simply turning the power of your imagination inwards for the health and healing of your own body. When you start directing your images in this way, you will have achieved a sense of control in your life and with managing your stress.

Magic Carpet Ride

The imagery script below, *Magic Carpet Ride*, is for general relaxation, the skill on which you are working. This exercise will teach you how to take a little vacation in your mind without ever leaving your living room. In subsequent chapters you will be using the tool of imagery in other ways, such as seeing specific muscles relax or your arteries dilate.

The Magic Carpet Ride Script

As you prepare yourself for this exercise, make sure that you will be comfortable and warm and that you will not be interrupted for the next 25 minutes. Begin by focusing your awareness on your breathing…breathing a deep, slow, conscious breath, holding for a moment after the inhalation, and then exhaling fully and completely. Allow yourself to continue to breathe slowly and naturally throughout this exercise.

Imagine that with every breath you can simply breathe away any tension or anxiety and allow yourself to relax more and more. As you continue to breathe slowly and naturally, imagine that you are watching any thoughts or memories that are running through your consciousness…seeing them from a distance…

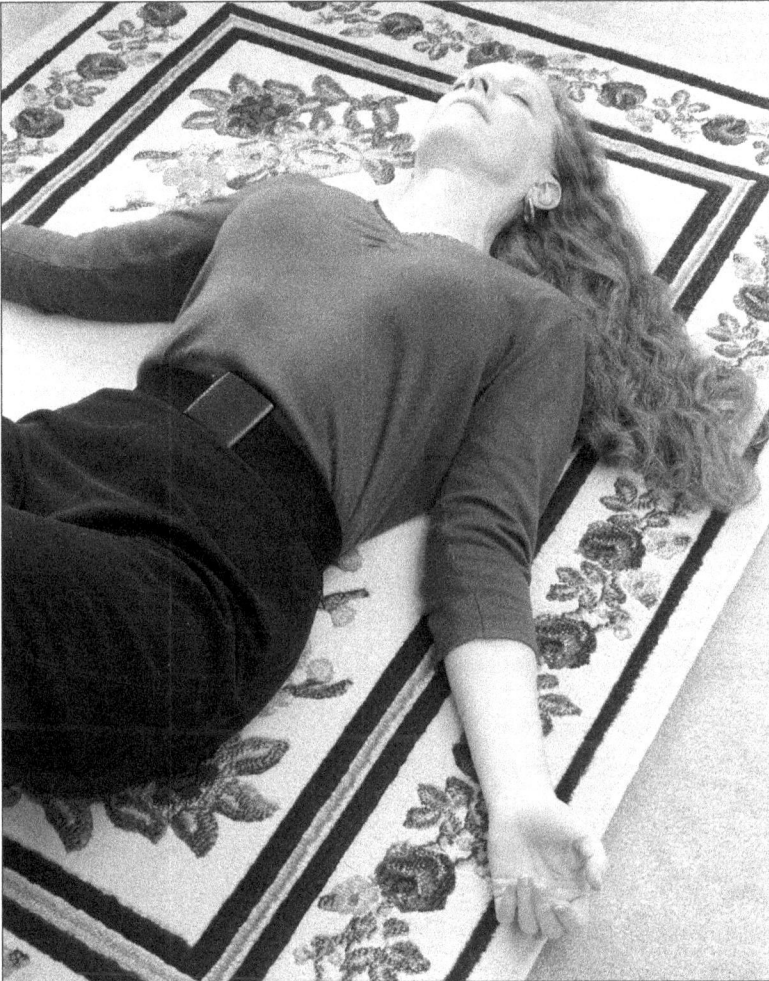

FIGURE 5.1
Preparing for Magic Carpet Ride imagery.

being fully aware of them without clinging to any of them…without letting them run you or control your life…just watching them as they float on by.

Now, focusing on your body…let yourself drift deeper into calm and total relaxation as you relax all the muscles in your legs and feet…feel the heaviness increasing here as the muscles relax, loose and limp. Now relax the muscles in your arms and hands…allowing the surface you are lying on to support the arms and hands…feel the heaviness here. Now moving your awareness to your neck and shoulders…allow these muscles to relax…make sure your neck is comfortable, and feel your head sinking into whatever surface you are lying on. Imagine a wave of relaxation moving through your body…it starts at your feet and moves slowly upwards, relaxing any place that may still be holding tension…moving through the legs, the torso and arms, the neck and the head…feel and imagine this wave of relaxation calming your body and stilling your mind.

Imagine now that you are in a meadow on a beautiful, warm spring day. The sky is clear and blue. The grass is green. As you look around, you notice all the colors and the visual details (pause)…and you hear the birds and the sound of the creek nearby…you smell the fresh spring air as you take a deep and full breath. You are alone, and you feel very much at peace…you know intuitively that you are safe…and protected from any distraction or intrusion. You find a very comfortable place in the meadow, and you go and lie down.

You notice that you are lying on a carpet. It is a magic carpet…a carpet that can take you wherever you want to go. As you lie there on the carpet, you notice how the carpet feels against your skin. You notice the colors and the patterns in the carpet. The carpet slowly begins to rise…just a little bit off the ground…and you begin to experience a pleasant floating sensation. The carpet begins to rise a little higher. You feel very safe and secure, and you know that you have complete control over your magic carpet. You can travel close to the ground…or go very high if you wish. You can travel slow or fast…whatever you choose.

You are free to travel anywhere you would like to go. Perhaps you would like to go to some special place you haven't been to before…or someplace you have been to that you want to return…maybe you would like to visit a friend or relative whom you are close to but haven't seen in a while…or maybe you just want to get some perspective on your life and surroundings. Take a few moments now to travel on your magic carpet…going wherever you wish to go. Be aware of all that you see, smell, hear and feel…being aware of all your senses as you travel. Have a peaceful and joy-filled journey as you travel now…(pause for a few minutes).

Take a moment to do whatever you need to do to feel complete with your journey for now (pause for 30 seconds)…. Find yourself again on your magic carpet now, returning to your point of departure…knowing that you can travel this way anytime you wish…going wherever you wish to go…but for now you return to the beautiful and peaceful meadow…and you very gently land your magic carpet where you began your journey. You will remember and cherish any special moments you had on your trip. You will remember just as much as you need to, and you know that the deeper part of you remembers everything you experienced on this beautiful journey.

If you are about to go to sleep now, you will fall asleep easily and effortlessly…sleeping well throughout the night…and you will wake up feeling refreshed and alert. If you are about to get up and continue on with your day, say to yourself, "I am refreshed and completely alert. I am refreshed and completely alert. I am refreshed and completely alert."…and as you are ready, you may gently open your eyes.

More Imagery Ideas

Whatever you can do to reduce your stress, which in turn calms your nervous system, will help improve your health. Here are just a few imagery ideas to help you feel more calm, safe and positive.

1. After a stressful day, I like to get in the shower and imagine that I am washing off all the stress and tension, which washes down the drain with the water. I imagine the stress coming out of my pores and being washed away. Whatever the situation, I find this helpful to let go of the day's tensions.

2. I like to imagine when I breathe that I am breathing in the qualities I choose to have more of in my life, and when I exhale I am breathing out those qualities I choose to have less of in my life. For example, I inhale peace and exhale anxiety; I inhale acceptance and exhale judgment; I inhale relaxation and exhale tension. You might want to make a list of the qualities you choose to have more of and the ones you choose to release.

3. When I want to clear my energy and/or create protection around me, I use this imagery technique. Sit in a comfortable position with your back straight and eyes closed. Imagine a golden light (you might see the sun to help you visualize the light) moving up from the base of your spine through the top of your head. The light comes out, and then it showers down all sides of your body, about six inches to a foot from your physical body, like a fountain of light. Keep circulating this light–up through the spine and then showering down–until you feel clear, safe and protected. When you feel complete, close off the imaginary place where the light went out of your head and imagine now that your entire body is filling with this golden light. It is a healing light, and every cell is able to absorb it.

Practice

1. Record the *Magic Carpet Ride* script and use it in place of, or in addition to, the deep relaxation tape. It is good to have a few tapes so that you don't get bored with one and lose your focus. Also, some people are naturally more attuned to imagery and will enjoy this one more. As with the body relaxation tape, you may record it with or without music in the background. If you would prefer to order this CD already recorded, simply go to

the website listed at the bottom of this page and you will find it available in the website store.

2. Practice your imagery skills on a daily basis. This will help you to develop the skill of directed imagery. You can play with some of the shorter imagery exercises listed above or make up your own. For example, you might imagine that everyone you see is wearing a pink hat, or imagine what you would feel like if you had a million dollars. Imagine whatever you like as long as it is filled with positive and constructive images. Learn to direct your imagination to create what you want. The more you use your imagination, the better you will become at this skill. This will help you later on with imagining your muscles relaxing and imagining your blood flow increasing. These may seem like silly exercises, but you will be able to use this powerful skill to your benefit as you move through this program. With the technique of imagery, just as with proper breathing and deep relaxation, you can shift the ANS back into a place of balance.

3. Are you staying on track with your stress calendar, breathing exercises, use of cue dots and practice of your autogenic (deep relaxation) exercise?

4

Relax Specific Muscles

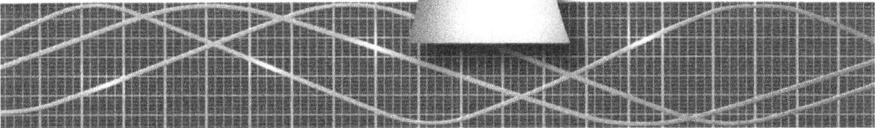

Reducing Muscle Tension

When the body perceives danger or stress, the muscles tense up. You may recall that during the fight-or-flight response, the body is preparing to fight off or flee the perceived danger. This physiological response occurs in reaction to psychological threats as well as physical dangers.

In biofeedback one of the physiological responses we measure is muscle tension. Muscle tension is measured by using a surface EMG (electromyogram). The muscle tension in any surface skeletal muscle can be measured in microvolts. Every muscle has a normal level of tension that is considered optimal for it. More muscle tension than this normal level can cause various physical problems, including headaches, backaches, and neck pain. Biofeedback therapists teach their patients how to bring the muscle tension in various parts of the body to normal to eliminate the symptoms.

In this step of the program you will be learning how to relax specific muscles in the upper body. It is essential that you not skip Lessons 6 and 7 on the shoulders and the neck. Because every animal, including the human variety, has an unconscious instinct to protect the throat, and because we are living in a fast-paced society during tense times, I can practically guarantee that the tension in your neck and shoulders is above normal. As I have mentioned previously, the lessons on jaw tension and eyestrain are optional, depending on how you answered the stress questionnaire. However, if you have any doubt as to whether you have excess muscle tension in the jaw or eye areas, it is better to do those lessons as well.

Remember that you do not need to feel aches, pain or stiffness in your muscles for the tension to be above normal. I once treated a teenage girl for migraines and measured the muscle tension on the top of her shoulders. Normal for the top of the shoulders is approximately 1.5 microvolts or less. Her readings were at 15.0 microvolts, or 10 times normal. Yet during the initial evaluation, she had reported not being aware of any tension or stiffness in her shoulders. You can imagine her surprise when she saw how high her muscle tension was!

Typically, I find that people with muscle tension that is three to five times normal experience pain from that tension. The pain could be in the head, neck, back, jaw, shoulders, or elsewhere in the body. If you follow the lessons in Step 4 very carefully, you can be assured that your muscle tension will drop down to normal or very close to normal. You do not need to be hooked up to biofeedback instruments to know that. If you are curious and do want your muscle tension measured in any of these areas, you can find a certified biofeedback therapist in your area by going to www.BCIA.org.

The Shoulders

Meet Your Trapezius Muscle

The trapezius muscle is a very large muscle that attaches at the base of the skull, goes down to the tips of the shoulders and about halfway down the back (see fig. 6.1). This is usually the first muscle to contract when a person perceives a threat. This is a key muscle for everyone to learn how to relax.

In this chapter, you will be given four tools to help bring shoulder tension to normal:

1. Imagery exercises designed specifically for relaxing shoulder tension;

2. A series of shoulder-muscle exercises to be practiced daily;

3. Posture awareness and correction information;

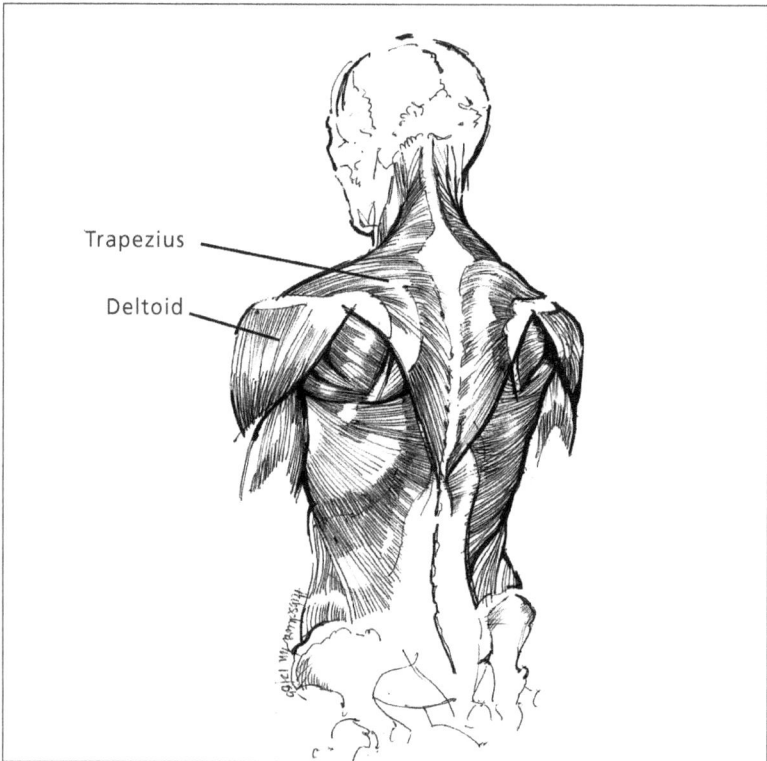

FIGURE 6.1 — The trapezius muscle is very tight in most people.

4. An explanation of the psycho-emotional aspects of the
   shoulders designed to lead to release of muscle tension here.

Imagery for Releasing Muscle Tension in the Shoulders

You may recall that imagery is a very powerful tool to use for
releasing tension from the body. Below are some imagery ideas I use

with patients for muscle relaxation of the shoulder area. Use these and also feel free to make up your own.

1. **Imagine strings.** It is very effective to use an image of a string on the top of the head gently lifting upwards to straighten and lengthen the spine. When the spine is supporting the body, the muscles will not have to work as hard to hold your body erect. Then the muscles can relax. Imagine a feeling of lightness in your body and lengthening in the spine as the string lifts upwards.

   I recall using this image during a seniors yoga class I was teaching. There were about 30 people aged 65 to 85 sitting in a circle with their eyes closed. They were all slouched over, as we tend to do when we age. When I asked them to imagine this string lifting upwards from the head, they all immediately straightened up through the spine and looked decades younger with this one simple image. It was a beautiful sight to see!

   Another string image to use is visualizing a string lifting up from the center of the chest. This lifts the ribcage and opens the breathing. It also helps to lengthen the spine.

2. **Increase the blood flow and circulation in the muscle itself.** When a muscle becomes very tight, as mentioned earlier, the blood cannot circulate freely in the muscle tissue. This can cause aches, pain, tension or discomfort in the muscle. Using your imagination, bathe the shoulder area with blood and oxygen. You might see a literal picture of the muscle and see the blood flowing there. Or try imagining a feeling of warmth there as you increase the blood flow in your shoulder area. Experiment with visualizing warm colors, such as orange, gold

or red, swirling around this area to increase the warmth and circulation.

3. **Imagine little lead weights.** Another effective tool for shoulder relaxation is to imagine little lead weights dangling from the tips of your elbows. Feel the gentle pulling and dropping of the upper arms and shoulders. Notice the sensation of heaviness as the arms and shoulders become more relaxed.

Exercises for Releasing Shoulder Tension

In all of these exercises, find the place where you feel a good stretch and release of muscle tension *without straining*. Breathe deeply as you hold these stretches, and imagine that you are sending oxygen and blood to the muscle that is being stretched. Remember, tight muscles are deprived of blood and oxygen. Strive to find a place of comfort and ease as you stretch.

I always tell people that it is better to err on the side of caution than to overdo it when first learning proper stretching. However, no matter how many times I say this, I occasionally have someone who believes in the "no pain, no gain" theory. Please forget that theory here! Be gentle. Breathe, relax and take your time, and you will be amazed how quickly your muscles will loosen up.

Caution: You should not feel any pain during or after any of the exercises presented in this book. If you do feel pain, immediately release the exercise. The exercises should feel good. Strive to find a place of pleasure and relaxation in your body as you move. If you have an injury in any of the areas affected by these exercises, have an osteopath or chiropractor guide you through the exercises and assist you in finding the ones you can do and the ones you should avoid.

Some of these exercises can be done either sitting or standing. If you are standing while doing any of them, be sure that your feet are two or three feet apart and that you are relaxed through the knees. Feel and imagine a solid base through your legs supporting you. You might imagine roots growing out of the bottoms of your feet that go deep into the earth.

All of the following exercises will release tension in slightly different areas of the shoulders. Do them all if you can.

1. **Shoulder rolls** – This exercise can be done either standing or sitting. The spine should be erect. You might imagine a string on the top of your head gently lifting upwards as your spine lengthens (fig. 6.2). Begin to roll the shoulders, first bringing them forward (fig. 6.3), then up towards the ears (fig. 6.4), then

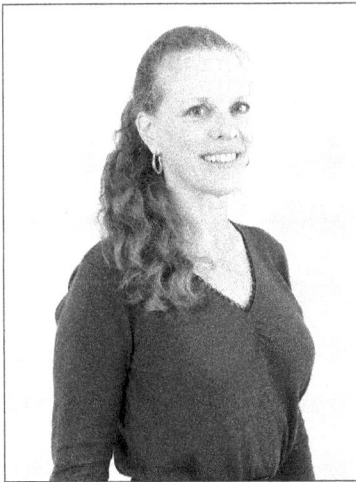

FIGURE 6.2
Shoulder rolls—sitting straight and tall.

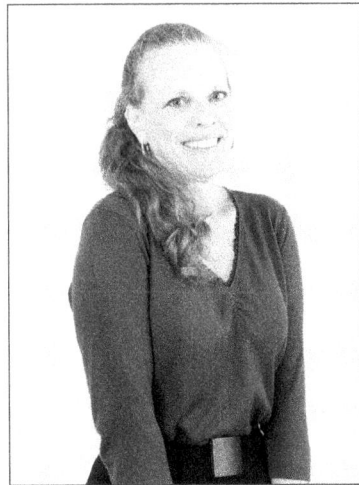

FIGURE 6.3
Shoulder rolls—bringing shoulders forward.

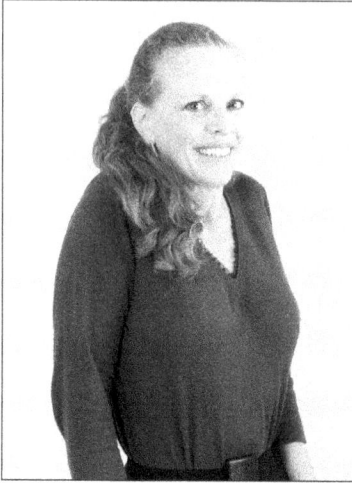

FIGURE 6.4
Shoulder rolls—up towards ears.

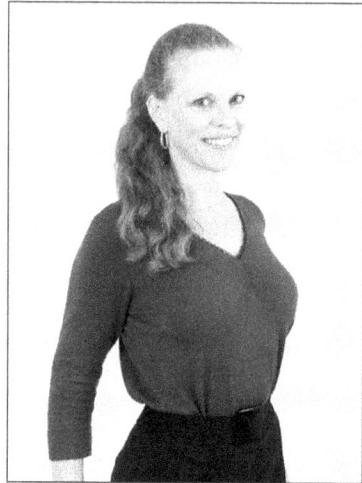

FIGURE 6.5
Shoulder rolls—back and opening chest.

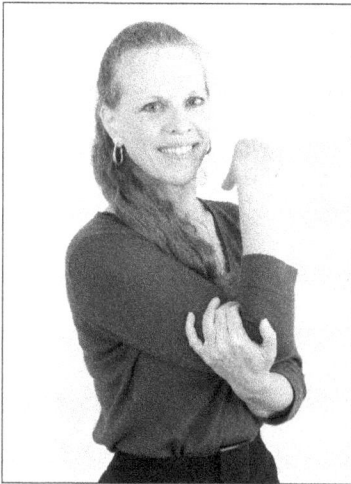

FIGURE 6.6
Shoulder release.

back, opening through the chest (fig. 6.5), and finally down again. Repeat three or four more times. Then, reverse the direction and make four or five more circles.

2. Shoulder release – This exercise can be done either standing or sitting. Bring one arm in front of the chest. Take hold near the elbow with the opposite hand. Gently pull the elbow towards the chest (fig. 6.6). Hold for 10 to 15 seconds. Then release and change sides.

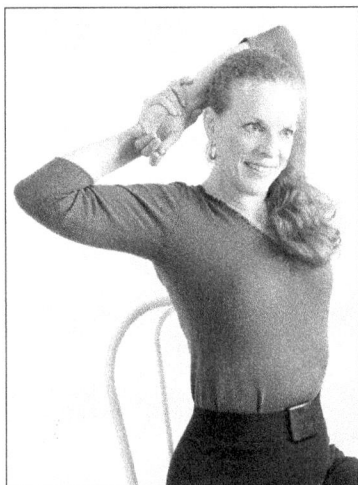

FIGURE 6.7
Shoulder stretch.

3. Shoulder stretch – This exercise can be done either standing or sitting. Bring one arm above the head. Bending at the elbow let the lower part of that arm drop behind the head. Now take hold of that wrist with the opposite hand. Gently pull down until you feel a comfortable stretch (fig. 6.7). Your head might need to come forward a bit. Find the place where you feel a good release of tension without straining, and hold for 10 to 15 seconds. Release and do the other side.

4. **Full arm circles** – This exercise is done in a standing position. Check to see that your spine is straight and tall. Relax slightly through the knees, being sure that your knees are not locked (fig. 6.8). Move with the breath. Inhaling, bring the right arm forward (fig. 6.9) and then up towards the ceiling, stretching as if you wanted to touch the ceiling (fig. 6.10). Exhaling, bring the arm down behind you as you continue the circle (fig. 6.11), and then bring the arm down by your side as you complete the exhalation. As you circle the right arm, keep the left arm and shoulder fully relaxed, imagining a feeling of heaviness here. Do two more full arm circles in this direction with the right arm. Reverse and do three circles in the opposite direction with the right arm, remembering to move with the breath. Then do the circles, first forward then backward, with your left arm.

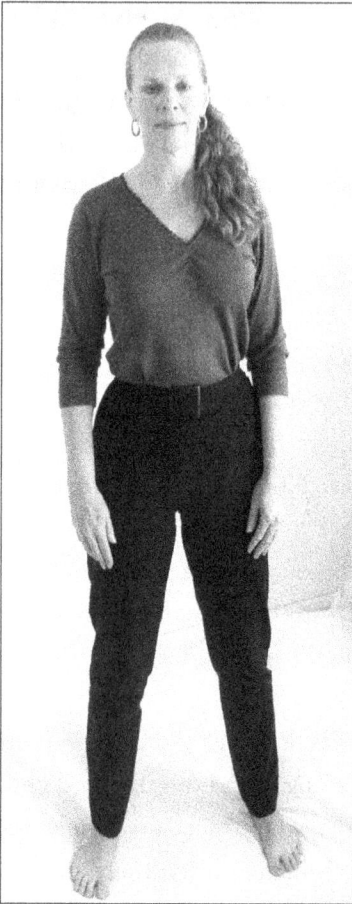

FIGURE 6.8
Preparing for full arm circles.

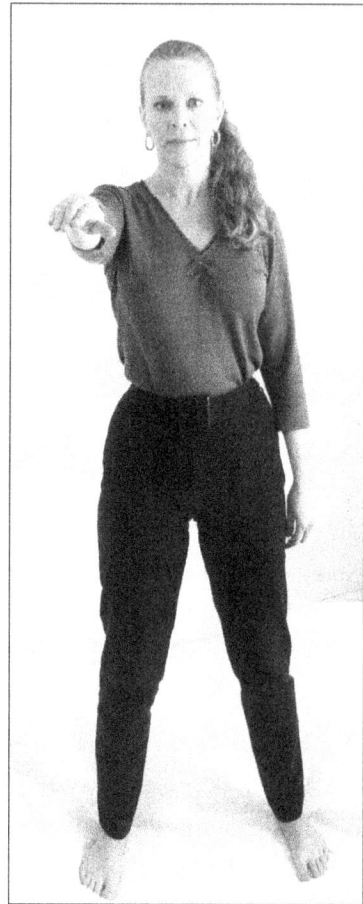

FIGURE 6.9
Full arm circles—arm forward.

5. **Trapezius stretch** – Sit with your spine straight and tall. Let the chin drop down towards the chest, keeping the shoulders back and down. Now interlace your hands and place them on the back of the head (fig. 6.12). Let the elbows gently drop down as your arms relax. Allow the weight of your arms to increase the stretch without forcing. Add as much weight as you

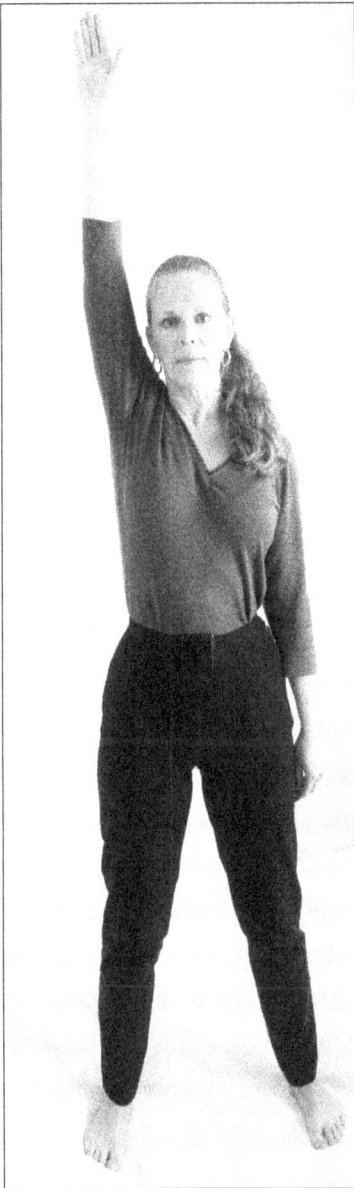

FIGURE 6.10

Full arm circles—reaching towards ceiling.

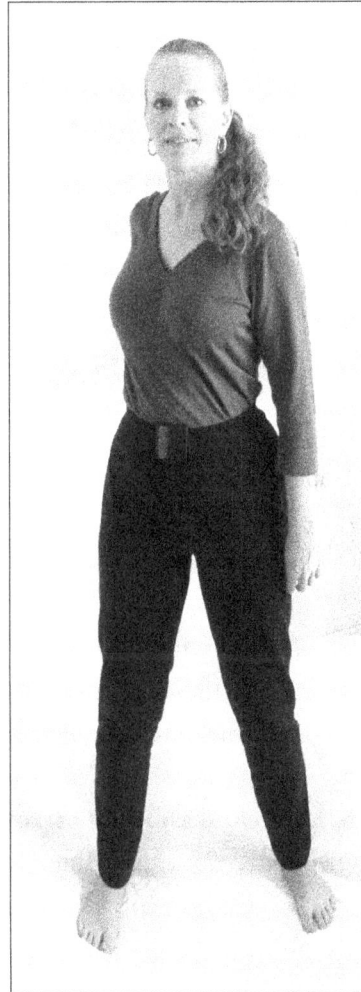

FIGURE 6.11

Full arm circles—arm to the back.

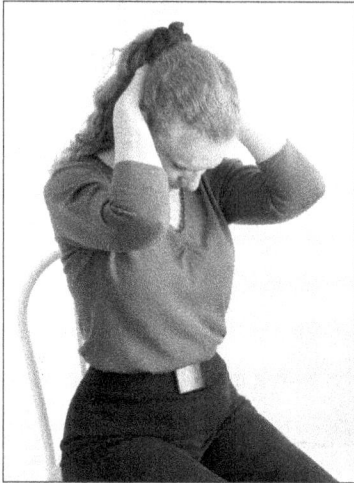

FIGURE 6.12
Trapezius stretch.

can *comfortably*. Initially, you might not put the full weight of your arms onto the back of your head. Hold for a few moments as you breathe the full, deep diaphragmatic breath. Then slowly and gently turn your head to the right with the weight still on the back of your head. Pause if you like. Then slowly roll the chin back towards the chest before turning the head to the left. Go back and forth a few times. Bring the head to the center, release the arms down and then roll the head up one vertebra at a time, imagining the vertebrae stacking in perfect alignment as you roll the head up. This is a wonderful stretch for the entire trapezius muscle. You will feel it first in the area of the muscle where you are most tense. Notice where you feel it the most. Is it in your shoulders, neck or upper back?

6. **Arm and shoulder stretch** – This exercise can be done either standing or sitting. Interlace your fingers, turning the palms out with the arms straight. Bring the arms up as far as you comfortably can (fig. 6.13). Eventually you will be able to bring the arms straight up by the ears. Hold the stretch for 10 to 15 seconds while you breathe diaphragmatically. Then release the arms down and unlace the fingers. Shake the wrists and hands. There is one variation that people often like. In this variation you move the arms up with the inhalation and down with the exhalation without pausing to hold the stretch. If you prefer movement

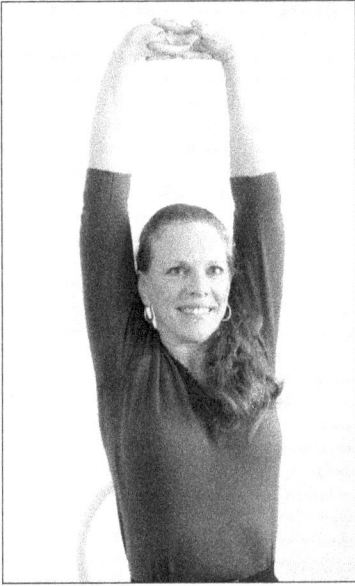

FIGURE 6.13
Arm and shoulder stretch.

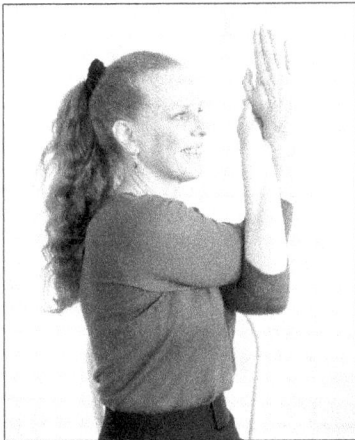

FIGURE 6.14
Twisty arms—with palms
together.

to holding the arms still, try this variation.

7. Twisty arms – This exercise can be done either standing or sitting. I recommend that you work with this exercise while sitting at first and then advance to the standing variation if it is appropriate for you. Sitting with the spine straight and tall, bring the arms in front of the chest with the right elbow over the left. Twist the arms while bending at the elbows and bring the palms of the hands together (fig. 6.14). If the palms do not comfortably come together simply bring them as close as possible. Hold this pose for a moment as you imagine the string lifting upward from the head and the shoulders dropping down. Now inhale slowly as you turn your head to look over the right shoulder (fig. 6.15). Pause. Exhale, bringing the head back to center. Inhaling, turn to look over the left shoulder. Pause. Exhale and return the head slowly to center. Now, with the next

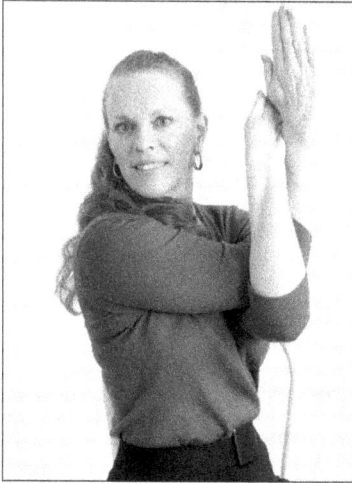

FIGURE 6.15
Twisty arms—looking over shoulder.

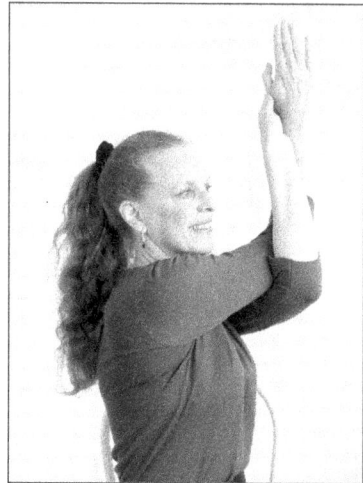

FIGURE 6.16
Twisty arms—bringing arms up.

inhalation bring the arms up with the arms still twisted (fig. 6.16). Pause with the arms up as you hold the inhalation. Exhale as you bring the elbows down. Begin to lean the torso forward, imagining there is a hinge in the hips and the back is straight as you come forward. When you can no longer keep the back straight begin to let it round, dropping the head and letting the shoulders drop while you continue to keep the arms twisted (fig. 6.17). Be sure there is no tension or holding in the neck. Let the muscles go loose and limp while you relax in the pose. Breathe deeply and slowly. Relax in this pose as long as you like. When you come up, roll up by stacking one vertebra at a time starting at the base of the spine. When you have returned to a sitting position, inhale and bring the arms up, noticing how much higher they go up this time. Exhale, bringing the arms back down. Untwist the arms and shake out the wrists and hands. Then repeat on the other side. This exercise is wonderful for releas-

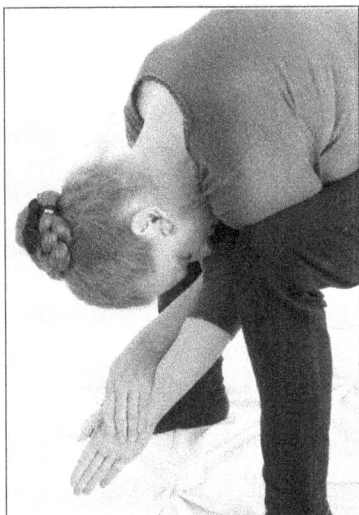

FIGURE 6.17
Twisty arms—leaning forward.

ing muscle tension in the upper back, especially between the shoulder blades.

Twisty arms – standing variation. *Caution: If you have low back problems, do the sitting variation only.* Stand with the feet about three feet apart and bent slightly at the knees. Follow the series of moves listed above in the sitting twisty arms exercise. As you hang forward, be sure to stay loose and limp through the back, neck and shoulders. As you are hanging you can sway the torso from right to left slowly if you like. In this variation you will be releasing tension from your entire back. When returning to the standing pose, bend even more at the knees. This is to protect your low back from muscle strain. Roll up, stacking the vertebrae, and continue with the moves as listed above.

Correcting Your Posture to Reduce Shoulder Tension

If your posture is poor, your muscles work hard to hold your body erect. The muscles in the back and neck become extremely tense when they are doing the work that the spine was meant to do. This excess tension contributes to stress in the body by tightening on the arteries and constricting blood flow.

There is a natural curvature in the spine that creates a cushioning effect as a person walks. The spine should be curved in the lumbar region and in the cervical, or neck, region. In these areas the spine should curve inward, creating *lordotic* curves. The curve in the thoracic spine is *kyphotic*, or outward. When these natural curves are thrown off due to poor posture, the back and shoulder muscles have to work very hard, which can lead to their becoming extremely tense. Remember, when the posture is correct, the spine will do most of the work of holding the body up so the muscles don't have to work as hard.

Chairs without lumbar support can cause the muscles in the upper back, neck and shoulders to work excessively hard. Often we sit in chairs that have totally straight backs. This means the lumbar part of the spine is held straight as it fits into the chair. The result is that the entire spine gets thrown out of its natural curve, and the muscles start to tense. And to make matters worse, with our sedentary lifestyle most people spend an excessive amount of time sitting at home, at work, and in the car.

When working on muscle tension in the shoulders, I find that adding lumbar support is the single most important thing to correct posture and reduce back and neck tension (fig. 6.18). It is crucial that you have good lumbar support while sitting, and it is simple to make this correction. Often a little pillow in the lumbar area will suffice.

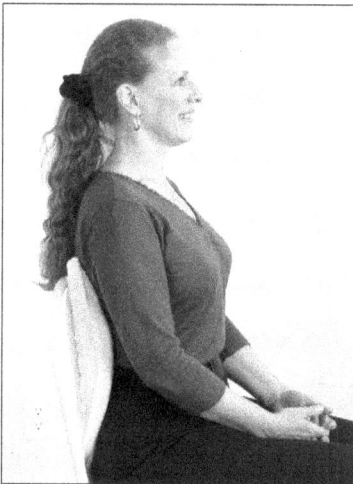

FIGURE 6.18

Proper lumbar support to relax back, neck and shoulder muscles.

Specifically designed lumbar support pillows are available as well. In my experience, stores that specialize in back-care products will often let you take several lumbar supports to your car so that you can see which works best in your car and what feels the best to your body.

If your work requires you to sit at a computer for many hours during the day, it would be well worth your time and money to have a complete ergonomic evaluation of your workstation. Many very serious conditions can develop as a result of repetitive strain on certain muscles or tendons. The human body is not designed to be sitting all day; it is designed to be in motion. It is critical that you use the body as efficiently as possible if you must spend hours sitting each day.

Psycho-Emotional Aspects of Shoulder Tension

Do you feel like you "carry the weight of the world" on your shoulders? If you do, you are carrying a lot of weight and your shoulders will reflect this by being very tense. Remind yourself that you are not responsible for the whole world. Take care of what is close at hand. People who are overly responsible tend to be highly stressed at the expense of their own health. See if you can begin to let go of some of the responsibilities that are not necessary for you to take on.

Have you ever noticed that the word "should" is in the word "shoulders"? When people hold chronic tension here, they often tell themselves that they "should" or "ought to" or "have to" do, or be, certain things. Replace the word "should" with "choose to" as it is much more empowering. For example, instead of saying to yourself, "I have to do the dishes" try saying, "I choose to do the dishes" or even "I choose *not* to do the dishes!" It is time to stop "shoulding" on yourself!

Practice

1. Do the shoulder exercises once a day or more. If you work at a computer, make a list of the exercises and do one exercise every half hour throughout the day. If you are not working at a desk, you can integrate the exercises into your exercise routine or do them separately. The most important thing is to do them every single day. Remember, you are creating new habits and a "new normal" level of tension in your shoulders. You need to be consistent.

   If you prefer to have a DVD of the exercises presented in this book so that you can see precisely how they are done and do them along with the verbal and visual instructions, go to the store at the website listed at the bottom of this page. The DVD entitled Stress Reduction Exercises includes the shoulder, neck, jaw and eye exercises found in this book.

2. Every time you see one of your cue dots, drop your shoulders, imagine that string lifting upwards from the top of your head, take a deep, full breath and say to yourself, "My shoulders are heavy and relaxed." Feel the heaviness in your shoulders as you consciously relax the muscles here.

3. Make sure you have adequate lumbar support in your car, at work and at home. Buy a good lumbar support pillow if necessary.

4. If you are a person who "shoulds" on yourself, begin to notice every time you use that word. You might be saying it aloud or it might be a thought that goes through your mind and is not expressed aloud. Either way, catch it and replace that thought

with a more empowering thought using the words, "I choose to…" or "I choose not to…."

5. Other things that can work well for releasing muscle tension in your shoulders and upper back include: hot Epsom salts bath (2 cups/tub), massage and yoga.

6. Are you continuing to practice your deep relaxation or the Magic Carpet Ride directed imagery tape daily? Are you practicing your diaphragmatic breathing daily for a minimum of 10 minutes? Are you continuing to track your stress induced symptoms and medication use? Are you beginning to notice that you are more relaxed overall and generally less reactive to situations that previously caused you to experience stress? If not, take more time with each new lesson and skill to gain some level of mastery before moving on.

Spend one full week working on relaxing the shoulder muscles before moving on to the next lesson. You need to create new habits by integrating shoulder awareness, shoulder exercises and posture correction into your life.

If you have followed the program carefully through the first six lessons and have practiced each skill to some level of mastery, you will be noticing a reduction in the frequency and severity of your stress and pain symptoms by now. Take a look at your stress charts to see exactly how much improvement you have made. Do you feel that you have achieved some level of mastery with the skills you've practiced to this point (diaphragmatic breathing, deep relaxation, and imagery)? Are they starting to become new habits? Are you beginning to notice more of a sense of peace and relaxation in your life?

The Neck

Know Your Neck from the Inside Out

In this lesson you will continue to release muscle tension from the trapezius muscle in addition to releasing tension from the other neck muscles. Several of the exercises in the previous chapter will have begun to loosen some of your neck tension by now. This chapter will teach you how to release any remaining excess tension from the front, back and sides of the neck. Remember, tension in the neck can constrict the blood flow to the head, which makes controlling neck tension critical for people suffering from migraines.

Take a look at the following illustration (fig. 7.1) to familiarize yourself with the neck muscles. It is helpful to have a visual image of what the muscles look like inside your body.

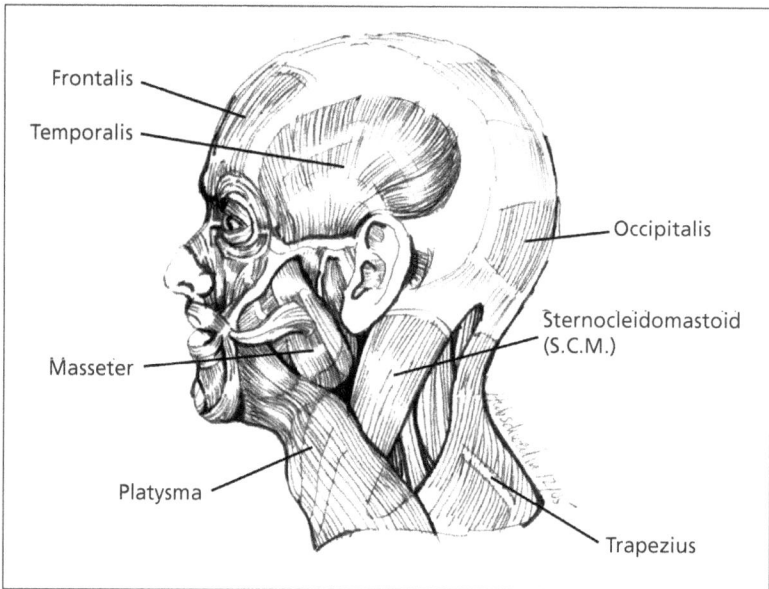

FIGURE 7.1

Relaxing the muscles in the neck and head is critical to avoid head–aches and neck pain.

In this chapter, you will learn how to release neck tension by:

1. Learning neck exercises to release muscle tension;

2. Understanding and healing the psycho-emotional aspects of the neck.

Neck Exercises

There are a few things to remember as you do these exercises. First, read the exercise directions completely before beginning the exercise. Next, remember to use the deep, diaphragmatic breathing the entire time you practice the exercises. Finally, don't overdo it.

Remember, it is better to be gentle until you know right where your limits are.

1. **Side stretch** – Sit comfortably in a chair with your spine straight and tall. Imagine those strings lifting upwards from the top of your head and the center of your chest. Breathe, relax and let the shoulders drop as you feel the heaviness in your shoulders. Now, slowly turn your head as you inhale and look over your right shoulder as far as you comfortably can. Feel the stretch in the neck as you hold for a moment (fig. 7.2). Then, with the exhalation release the head back to center. Inhale and turn your head to look over the left shoulder as far as you comfortably can. Pause, and with the exhalation release the head back to center. Move slowly and breathe deeply as you turn your head from right to left two more times in each direction.

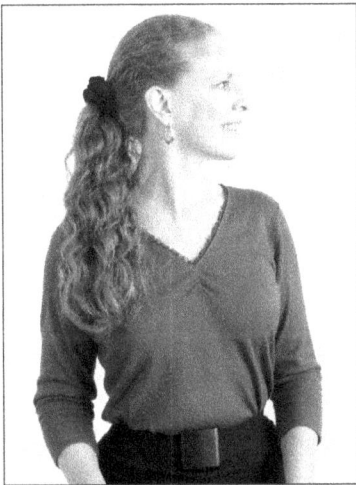

FIGURE 7.2

Neck stretch—looking over shoulder.

We turn our heads hundreds of times throughout the day and very often use the wrong muscles for the job. The sternocleidomastoid (SCM) muscles are the muscles that should work when you turn your head. Many people use their trapezius muscle. This poor muscle becomes so overworked! We use it to shoulder our stress and burdens, tense it when we are breathing wrong and then use it to turn the head. It is not surprising we carry excess tension in the trapezius.

As you turn your head from side to side, imagine that it is the SCM muscles that are turning the head (see illustration of the neck muscles in figure 7.1) rather than the trapezius muscle. While turning, imagine the shoulder muscles being very heavy and relaxed as if they cannot work to turn the head. If you feel the trapezius muscle working as you turn your head from side to side, try to keep it from working by not looking so far over your shoulders.

2. **Up-down exercise** – Again, make sure you are sitting comfortably with your spine straight and tall. Inhale and lift the chin up as you stretch the muscles in the front of your neck (fig. 7.3). Be sure not to drop the head back completely as you will compress the vertebrae. Pause for a moment as you hold the inhalation and feel the stretch in the front of the neck. As you exhale let the head slowly drop down bringing the chin to the chest while the

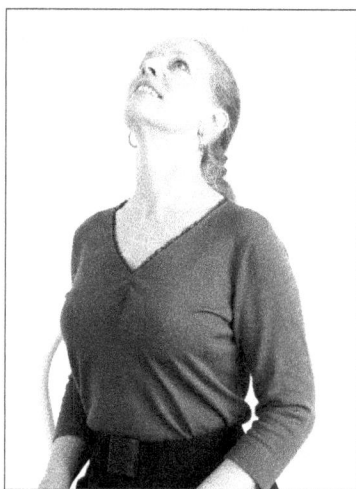

FIGURE 7.3
Lifting chin upwards—stretching front of neck.

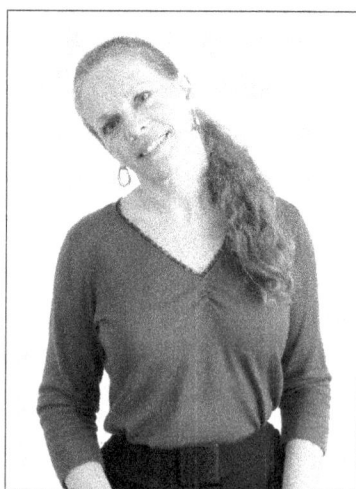

FIGURE 7.4
Neck stretch—ear towards shoulder.

shoulders remain back and down. Pause for a moment with the exhalation. Then inhale while bringing the head up and continue this up-down stretch for two more repetitions.

3. **Ear to shoulder stretch** – Sitting straight and tall, imagine the shoulders being heavy and relaxed, and at the same time imagine feeling little lead weights on the tips of your elbows. Now let the right ear begin to drop towards the right shoulder (fig. 7.4). Breathe deeply as you feel the stretch. Let the left shoulder drop and be heavy. Imagine that you are directing blood and oxygen to the muscles that are being stretched. Bring the head slowly back to center and then let the left ear drop towards the left shoulder, imagining the right shoulder being heavy and relaxed. Feel the stretch on the right side of the neck. Bring the head back to center and repeat two more times on each side.

4. **Diagonal neck stretch** – Turn your head slightly to the right. Exhale bringing the head forward while keeping the shoulders back and down. Now inhale bringing the head up and then back slightly stretching the left front side of your neck. As with the up-down stretch, do not let the head drop fully back. Instead, come to the point where you feel lengthening in your neck with no compression. Feel heaviness in your shoulders and arms. Pause for a moment with the head lifted upwards while holding the inhalation. Then exhale, releasing the head down, and continue for two more repetitions.

When your chin is hanging towards the right side of the chest for the third time, bring the right hand to the left shoulder and begin to massage the top of the shoulder, going as deep as you comfortably can. Remember to breathe the full, diaphragmatic breath. Massage the top of the shoulder fully and then let your

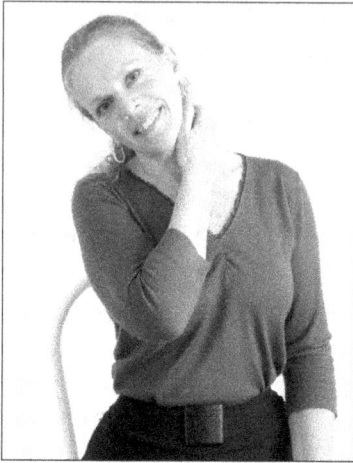

FIGURE 7.5

Massaging the neck.

hand move slowly up the left side of the neck massaging as you go (fig.7.5). Move to the base of the skull and massage there. The base of the skull is a good place to massage because this is where the trapezius attaches to the skull. When you have finished massaging this area, begin to let the hand move down the left side of the neck, massaging the muscle as your hand moves down, going all the way out to the tip of the left shoulder.

Notice if you feel any knots or lumps of tension in your shoulder or neck as you massage. If you do, you might want to pause at those tense spots and spend a little extra time there. This will bring extra blood and oxygen to the muscle and assist in releasing the muscle tension. When you have finished with this shoulder and neck massage on the left side, release your arm down and bring your head back to center. Pause for a moment to notice the difference between the right side and the left side. Then turn your head slightly to the left and do this entire series on the opposite side.

5. **Half circles** – While sitting straight and tall, let the right ear drop towards the right shoulder, remembering to keep the left shoulder down. Then roll the head forward, bringing the chin to the chest. Keep rolling the head until the left ear is above the left shoulder. Then lift the head back to center and make two more slow half circles in this direction. When the head comes

to center, reverse the direction and go three times slowly in the other direction.

Note: If you have whiplash or another neck injury that makes it difficult for you to lift the weight of your head up from the shoulder to the center position, try the following variation. While sitting straight and tall, drop the chin towards the chest with the shoulders back and down. Roll the right ear towards the right shoulder, and pause for a moment when the ear is above the shoulder. Then roll the head forward so the chin comes to the chest before rolling the head so that the left ear is above the left shoulder. Pause for a moment here. Continue rolling the head several times in this way. When you are ready to bring the head back up, roll the chin to the chest and roll the head up from this position, stacking the vertebrae one at a time as you roll up.

6. Standing Neck Stretch – While standing with your feet slightly apart, bring your hands behind your back and take hold of the left wrist with the right hand. Keep the shoulders back and down. While holding the left arm down with the right hand, begin to let the right ear drop towards the right shoulder (fig. 7.6). Notice the increased

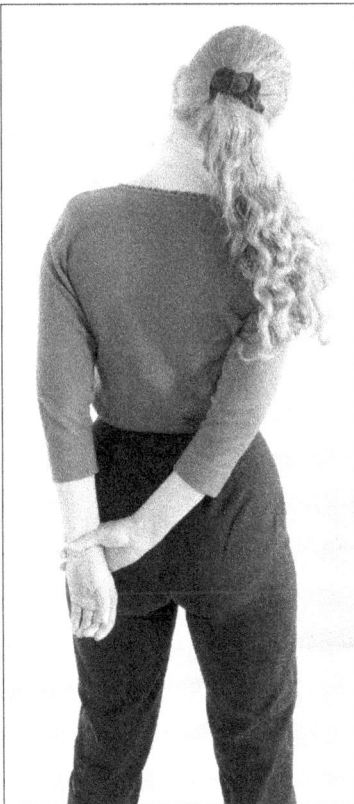

FIGURE 7.6
Standing neck stretch.

stretch as you hold the arm down (versus doing the ear to shoulder stretch above). Breathe deeply as you hold this stretch for a few breaths. Then release the stretch and bring the head slowly back to center. Now take hold of the right wrist with the left hand behind the back and drop the left ear towards the left shoulder. Repeat this exercise two more times on each side. If this stretch is too strenuous, stay with the ear-to-shoulder stretch above until your neck and shoulders have more flexibility. Then add this exercise to your routine.

Psycho-Emotional Aspects of Neck Tension

Have you ever used the phrase, "This is a pain in the neck!"? Earlier, we talked about the mind-body connection. When you say that something is a pain in the neck, pain can take hold there. Everything that happens in the mind is also manifested in the body. Even if you don't say something aloud but you think it, the thought will be felt, or embodied, in the physical. So it is important to be very aware of what you say to yourself.

In Step 5 you will learn more about the power of your thoughts. For now, if you are aware of anything in your life that you consider to be "a pain in the neck," first notice the thought. The thought might be about a person, situation, your job or anything that is bothering you. Then release that thought and replace it with a statement that is positive and believable. For example, you might say to yourself, "I am grateful for every situation and person in my life. I know that everything is here to help me to grow." Or make up whatever positive statement that works for you when this negative thought appears. This practice will actually help balance your nervous system and ease your nervous tension. Remember, it is essential to balance your nervous system in order to take control of the stress in your body.

Practice

1. Do the neck exercises presented in this lesson regularly. If you can fit the neck exercises and the shoulder exercises into your daily schedule, that would be ideal. If not, alternate these two sets of exercises, doing the neck exercises one day and the shoulder exercises the next day. Be sure to chart which exercises you do each day on your stress calendar. This will help you to stay on track.

2. Make a list of anything or anybody in your life that you consider to be a "pain in the neck." If it is possible to release these things or people from your life, you can choose to do that now. If they cannot be removed from your life, begin to reframe in your mind how you perceive these people or things. We will go into much greater detail in Step 5 on how to do this. For now, you can simply make some *positive* statement that works for you.

3. Are you staying on track with practicing your deep relaxation or Magic Carpet Ride tape daily? Are you doing conscious breathing? Are you still seeing your cue dots, or is it time to change the color? Are you recording on your stress chart daily? Are your shoulders and neck becoming more relaxed? Remember to stay on each lesson as long as necessary to establish what you've learned as a new habit before moving on to the next lesson.

Lesson

8

The Eyes

Eyestrain and Stress

Do your eyes ever feel strained? Do you wear glasses? Do your eyes get tired when reading or looking at the computer screen for an extended period of time? If you answered "yes" to any of these questions, this lesson is for you. When the eyes become strained you can start to feel tension in the head. Even if you are not aware of having eyestrain and you do not wear glasses, this is a good lesson for helping to prevent eyestrain and even the need to wear glasses.

Take a look at the following illustration (fig. 8.1). Notice the muscles that wrap around the eyes. Also notice the muscles that attach to the sides, the top and the bottom of the eyeball. These muscles need to be flexible and strong for optimal health of the eyes.

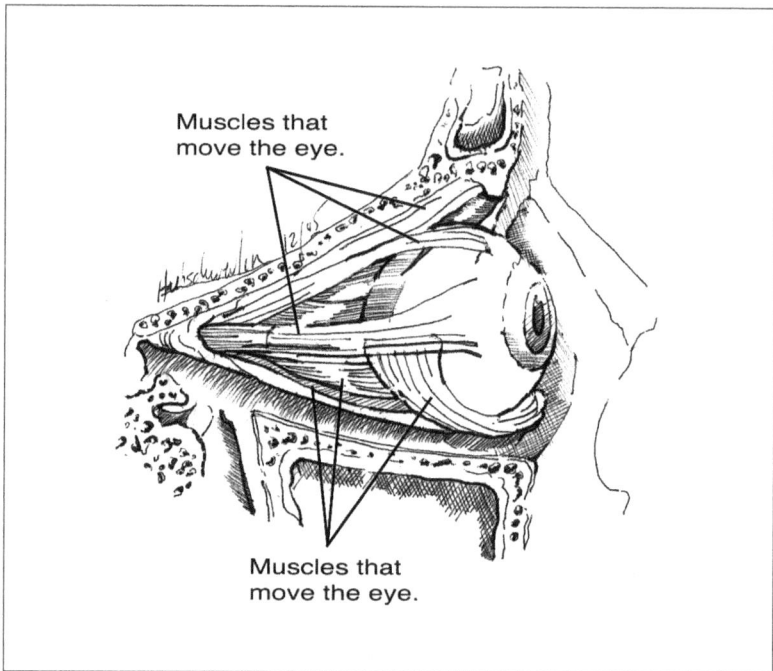

FIGURE 8.1—Tension in the eye muscles can contribute to head-aches or feeling tired.

If these muscles do not get exercise on a regular basis, they can lose their flexibility and become tight and constricted. When this happens, it can cause the eyeball to be pulled or pushed slightly out of shape. This can distort the lens of the eye, resulting in near-sightedness or farsightedness depending upon which direction the eyeball is distorted. Many people have had dramatic improvement with their eyesight by practicing these simple eye exercises on a daily basis. The exercises will also make your eyes stronger and less prone to eyestrain and the resulting tension in head and face muscles that can lead to headaches.

Eye Exercises

You might find it beneficial to make a tape of these eye exercises. If you choose to record the instructions, read aloud very slowly so that you will have time to do each exercise as you are hearing the instructions. The exercises will be much more relaxing if you do not need to stop to turn the tape off and on. If you have the DVD, *Beyond the Stress Mess Exercises,* you can do the eye exercises right along with the instruction provided.

The first time you do these exercises, start with three repetitions of each exercise. If your vision is not very blurred and your eye muscles do not feel overstretched at the end of this first session, then you can immediately increase the number of repetitions to five the next day. For most people, five repetitions of each will work well. However, as mentioned several times already, it is better to err on the side of caution than to overstretch or strain a muscle. If you wish to improve your eyesight in addition to releasing eyestrain, you should do the entire eye exercise series two times every day.

If you wear glasses, remove them before doing the exercises. Patients report that they successfully wear soft contact lenses while doing the exercises without discomfort.

Prepare yourself for these eye exercises by sitting in a comfortable position and allowing yourself ten minutes where you will not be disturbed. Notice the farthest point you can see in the distance. This is a point you will come back to; we will call it the *center point* or simply the *point.* At the end of each exercise you will come back to this center point. Notice whether your vision is blurry or clear each time you return to this point. It is natural to experience a slight amount of blurring. However, if your vision becomes extremely blurry, you may be overstretching your eye muscles. The muscles should not feel

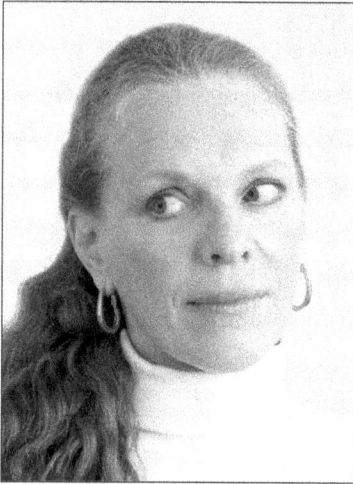

FIGURE 8.2
Eye exercises—side to side.

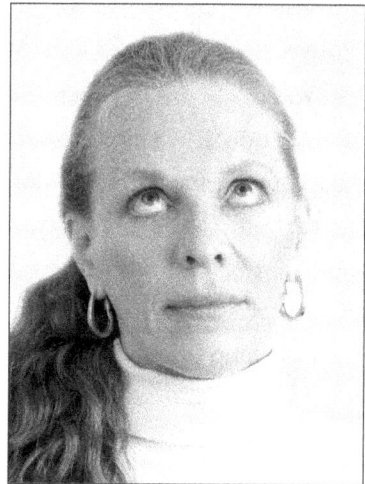

FIGURE 8.3
Eye exercises—up and down.

strained but pleasantly stretched. Blinking during these exercises is natural and serves to keep the eyeball moist.

1. **Side to side** – Sitting comfortably, begin by focusing on your center point. Now let your eyes move slowly to the right side without turning your head at all (fig. 8.2). Look as far as you comfortably can to the right, noticing the farthest point you see. Hold for a moment. Feel the stretch. Then release and bring the eyes slowly back to center, noticing every point along the way. Next, let the eyes move to the left side. Look as far as you can to the left as you hold the stretch for a moment. Release and let the eyes slowly come back to center. Do two more repetitions to each side. Notice whether you can look a tiny bit farther each time you look to the right or left. When your eyes come back to center after the third repetition, focus on your center point for a moment. Then close your eyes and let them rest for about ten seconds.

2. **Up-down exercise** – Open your eyes and focus on your center point. Now let the eyes move up towards the ceiling without moving the head at all (fig. 8.3). Notice the highest point you can see. Feel the stretch and hold. Then release and let the eyes move slowly downward as you notice every point along the way. Now look down without moving the head. Pause. Release and let the eyes begin to move back up. Continue the up-down eye exercise for two more repetitions. Then, when the eyes come back to center, focus on your point. Close your eyes and let them rest.

3. **Diagonals** – Open your eyes and focus on your point. Begin to let the eyes move slowly to the upper right, noticing the farthest point you can see (fig. 8.4). Stretch the eyes and hold. Release slowly down to center and then move to look to the lower left without moving the head. Notice the farthest point you see. Hold. Release the eyes, bringing them slowly back to center while noticing every point along the way. Continue with two more diagonal stretches in this direction. Then bring your eyes to center and focus on your point. Close your eyes and let them rest.

   Open your eyes. Now you will do diagonal stretches in the opposite directions. Start by moving your eyes to the upper left. Stretch. Pause. Release your eyes slowly back to center and let the eyes continue down until you are looking to the lower right. Notice the farthest point you can see. Hold while you feel the stretch. Release the eyes back to center. Do two more repetitions in this direction. When the eyes come back to center, focus on your center point. Now close your eyes and let them rest.

4. **Circles** – Open your eyes and focus on your point. Now let the eyes move up towards the ceiling, looking as high as you can without moving the head. Let the eyes begin to move in a clock-

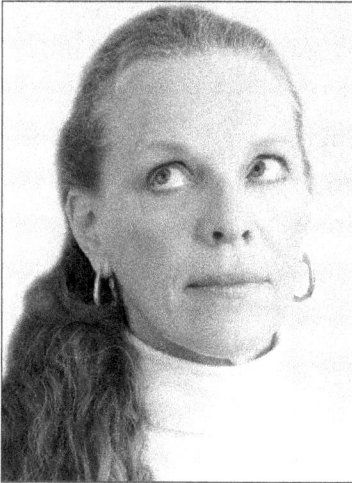

FIGURE 8.4
Eye exercises—diagonals.

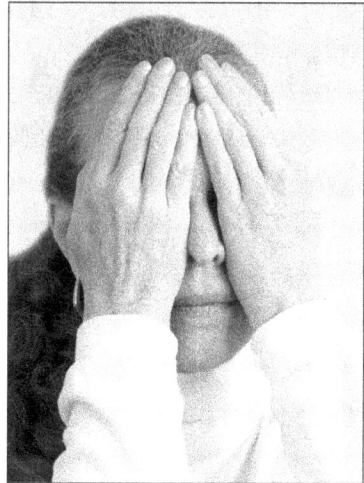

FIGURE 8.5
Eye exercises—palming.

wise direction–moving to one o'clock, two o'clock, three, four…
all the way to twelve o'clock. Bring the eyes back to center. Focus
on your point. Close the eyes and let them rest.

Now open your eyes. Focusing on your point, let the eyes
move back up to twelve o'clock. This time move in the other direction–eleven o'clock, ten o'clock, nine, eight…all the way back
to twelve o'clock. Bring the eyes back to center and focus on your
point. Close your eyes and let them rest.

5. **Palming** – With your eyes still closed, rub the palms of your
hands together until you create some heat. When the hands feel
hot, gently cup the palms of your hands over your eyes (fig. 8.5).
Feel the warmth penetrating the eye area. Imagine your eyes
relaxing as they absorb this warm feeling. With the hands still
cupped over the eyes so that no light shines through, imagine

total blackness. Notice whether you are able to see total blackness or there is some murkiness or color. This is an eye strengthening exercise. Very often it can take some time before people see total blackness. Hold for a few moments. Then, when you are ready, gently let the hands slide down away from your eyes, bringing the arms to a resting position. As you are ready, slowly open your eyes.

Practice

Practice the eye exercises as often as you can. Daily is ideal. If your schedule is too full to practice the shoulder exercises, neck exercises, and the eye exercises daily, rotate doing one series each day. Make a note on your stress chart of which exercises you do each day. This way, you will remember to stay on track and you won't forget ·any of the exercises.

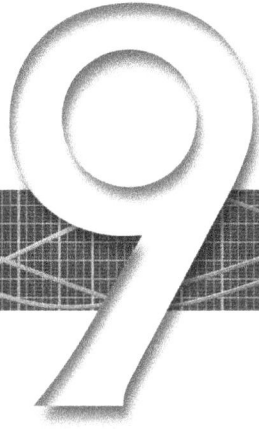

The Jaw

Say "Hello" to Your Jaw

Many people hold tension in their jaw. This tension can contribute to headaches, wearing of the teeth, and other problems which are easily avoidable. Sometimes people are aware when they clench or grind their teeth, and sometimes they are completely unaware that they are doing this. There are several questions you can ask yourself to determine if you hold tension in the jaw area.

- Does your jaw ever feel sore?
- Are your teeth wearing?
- Has your partner told you that you grind your teeth at night while you are sleeping?
- Are your teeth touching right now or are they slightly apart?

- Is your tongue relaxed and lying on the bottom of your mouth or is it holding tension and touching the roof of your mouth?
- Has your dentist told you that it looks like you grind your teeth, or has he/she recommended a night splint?
- Can you easily open your jaw to three finger widths without straining?
- Do you experience clicking or popping in your jaw?

If you answered yes to any of these questions, it would be beneficial for you to do this chapter.

There are many reasons people clench and/or grind their teeth. People often clench or grind when they are in physical pain. Repressing anger or frustration can lead to jaw tension. Holding back something you want to say can create tension here. Jaw problems often result from poor dental work. Additionally, motor vehicle accidents can throw the jaw out of alignment, creating temporomandibular joint, or T.M.J., disorders.

Dentists often prescribe night splints if they see that a person is clenching or grinding his or her teeth. These splints can be very effective in protecting the teeth from damage and wear. However, generally they do not get to the root of the problem, which is the contraction of the muscles in the T.M.J. area.

Look at the following illustration (fig. 9.1) and familiarize yourself with the bones and muscles in the T.M.J. area. Take particular notice of the masseter and pterygoid muscles as these are the muscles that generally constrict when people clench and/or grind. The masseter is the primary muscle used for chewing, talking and opening and closing the mouth in general. It is located directly under the surface of the skin. Notice that the pterygoid muscles are deeper

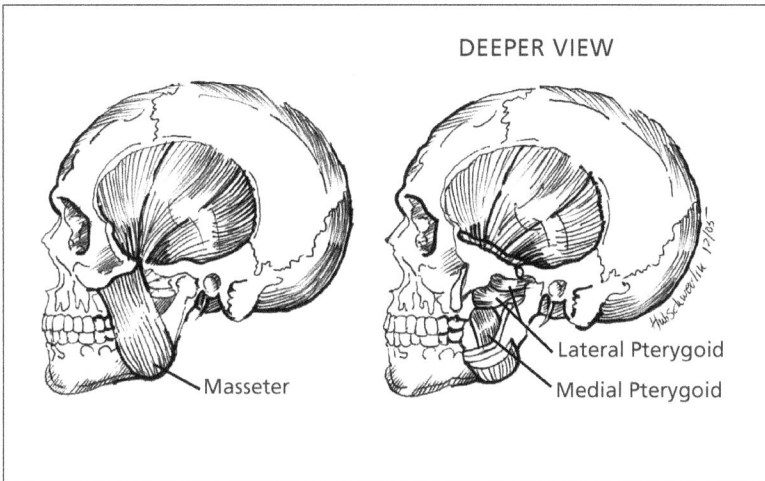

FIGURE 9.1—Clenching or grinding in the jaw can contribute to jaw pain, wearing of teeth, or headaches.

and can be felt from within the mouth. The second illustration shows these muscles.

Constriction in the masseter and pterygoid muscles creates not only jaw tension, but also increased muscle tension in the head by radiating into the temples. This causes the temporalis muscles to tighten. Excess muscle tension in the jaw area can be controlled.

Clenching or grinding can damage your teeth, creating the need for very expensive dental work. I had a patient once who told me he had more than ten thousand dollars' worth of dental work because of his clenching and grinding. This kind of situation is preventable. You simply need to become aware of the tension and then learn how to control it.

Relaxing the muscles in your jaw area is crucial to eliminating jaw pain, headaches, and preventing dental problems.

In this lesson you will learn how to:

1. Increase strength and flexibility of muscles in the jaw area by doing jaw exercises;
2. Communicate with your subconscious to stop clenching and/or grinding while sleeping;
3. Release tension from the pterygoid muscles;
4. Recognize and release psycho-emotional causes of jaw tension.

Jaw Exercises

The following exercises will help to make your jaw muscles both strong and flexible.

Again, remember to err on the side of caution when first doing these exercises. If you can only open your mouth one or two finger widths at this time, do not go to three finger widths until you are sure you are ready. You will be amazed how quickly these muscles will loosen up if you practice these exercises daily.

Build up slowly, especially if you hold a great deal of tension in the jaw. Start with half the repetitions that are suggested if you need to. Find the place where you feel the stretching and strengthening without overdoing it. Never deviate the jaw to one side. If the exercises create excessive soreness in the jaw area, again reduce the number of repetitions until you build your strength and flexibility. As you do the exercises, be sure to avoid any grating, clicking or popping noises in the jaw. If you experience any of these symptoms, see your dentist, chiropractor or osteopath for his or her guidance.

1. **Rhythmic Jaw Exercise** – Using a clock with a second hand, time yourself for one minute as you perform this exercise. Start

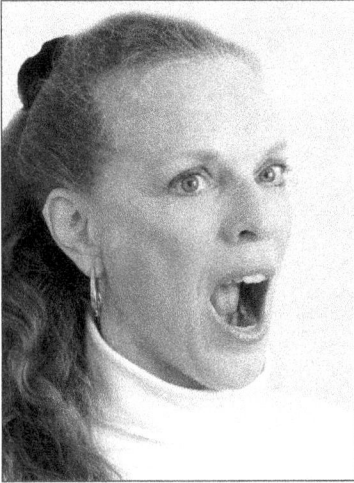

FIGURE 9.2
Rhythmic jaw exercise.

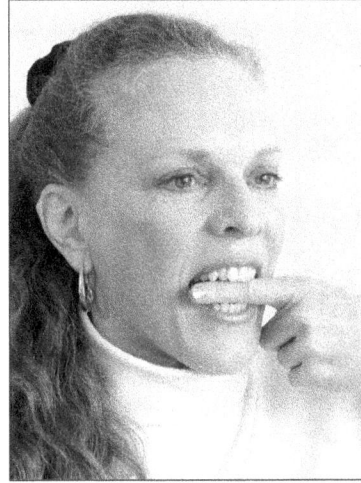

FIGURE 9.3
Jaw stretching—one finger.

with the jaw in the relaxed position with the teeth slightly apart. Open the jaw (straight up and down) about two finger widths (fig. 9.2) if you are able. Then close the jaw without biting the teeth together, bringing it to the resting position. Continue to open and close the mouth in this way in rapid succession for one minute.

2. **Jaw Stretching Exercise** – Place one finger between your teeth and let your teeth gently rest on your finger for 60 seconds as you use a clock with a second hand to time (fig. 9.3). Then remove the finger from the mouth, pause, and notice how the jaw feels. Rest for a moment. Now, if it is comfortable place two finger widths between your teeth and again gently rest the teeth on the fingers for 60 seconds (fig. 9.4). Remove the fingers and rest the jaw. Again, be aware of how the jaw feels. This may be where you

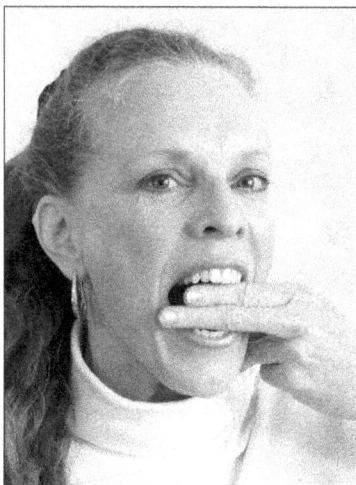

FIGURE 9.4
Jaw stretching—two fingers.

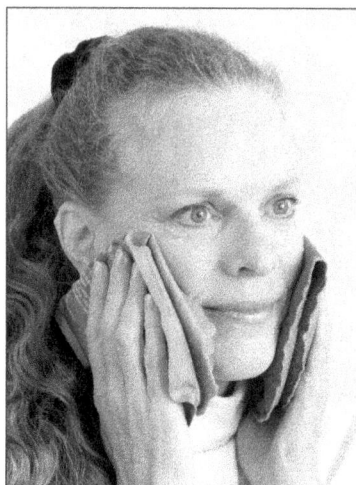

FIGURE 9.5
Applying ice to the T.M.J.

need to stop until your jaw area loosens. Do not attempt to go to three fingers between the teeth until it is comfortable and easy.

If the two-finger stretch feels like enough for now, pause for a moment in the resting position and become aware of how your jaw area feels. Then finish with an application of heat or ice on the T.M.J. area (fig. 9.5). Heat can feel very comforting to the muscles but can cause inflammation or irritation in some people. You might want to experiment with heat and ice at different times to determine which works best for you. Another option is to apply heat followed by ice. Keep the heat or ice on the jaw area for a couple of minutes or for as long as it feels comfortable to you.

If you can comfortably go to three fingers between the teeth (fig. 9.6), do that stretch for 60 seconds before applying the heat or ice.

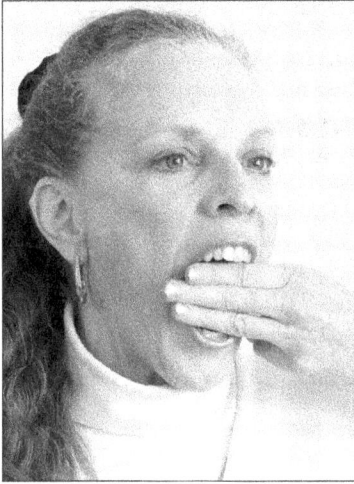

FIGURE 9.6
Jaw stretching—three fingers

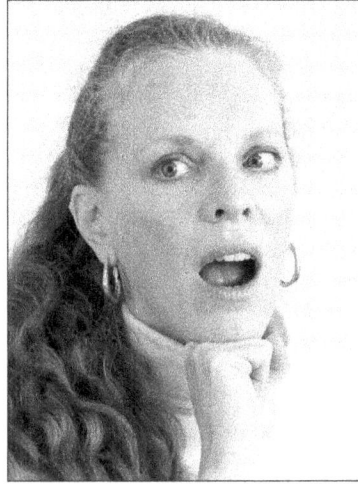

FIGURE 9.7
Jaw strengthening.

3. **Jaw Strengthening** – Start with your teeth slightly apart and make a fist with your hand. Rest your chin on the fist between the first and second fingers. Now push up gently with the fist against the chin while keeping the teeth apart. Next, open the mouth one to two finger widths while pressing the chin against the fist (fig. 9.7). Hold the fist and arm steady and strong. With the mouth open, hold to the count of ten. Feel the muscles being worked in the jaw area as you hold. Now, slowly bring the fist down away from the chin before closing the mouth so there is no pressure against the chin as you close. Repeat this exercise four more times for a total of five repetitions.

Pterygoid Massage

The pterygoid muscles are located inside the mouth near the T.M.J. (refer to fig. 9.1). Notice the medial and lateral pterygoid muscles. The most effective way to release tension from these muscles is by massaging the muscles. Prepare by washing your hands thoroughly or using latex gloves.

Going inside your mouth with your index finger (fig. 9.8), massage the pterygoid muscles moving in the direction of the muscle. Use a firm pressure. It will be easy to find these muscles if they hold any excess tension. They will be somewhat tender or sore as you rub. Massage for 30 to 60 seconds on each side. After removing your hand pause for a moment to notice how those muscles feel. They should feel just slightly tender from being worked. If they don't, try going a little bit deeper next time. Conversely, if they feel extremely sore use a softer pressure in the future.

If you are not sure that you are doing this correctly, you can have a chiropractor, a massage therapist or an osteopathic physician guide you through the pterygoid muscle massage.

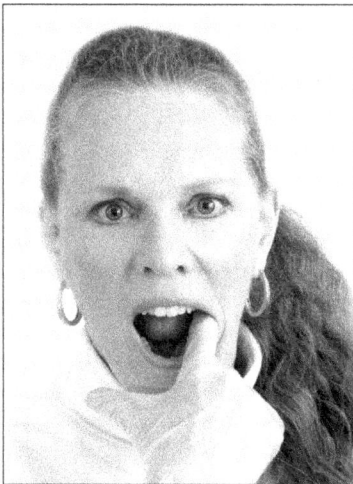

FIGURE 9.8
Ptergoid massage.

Jaw and Temple Massage

This is an effective and quick massage that you can do while at your desk or watching television. With your teeth apart, use your fingertips to massage firmly around the T.M.J. (fig. 9.9). Then let your fingertips move downwards and massage the muscles lower on the jaw using a firm pressure again. Finally, move your fingertips up to the temporalis muscle and massage here in a circular motion (fig. 9.10). You will notice this area feeling really good after just a couple minutes of massage.

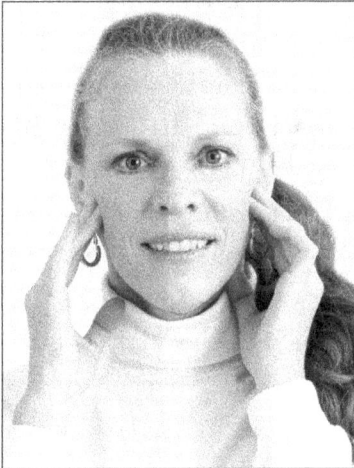

FIGURE 9.9
Massaging the T.M.J. area.

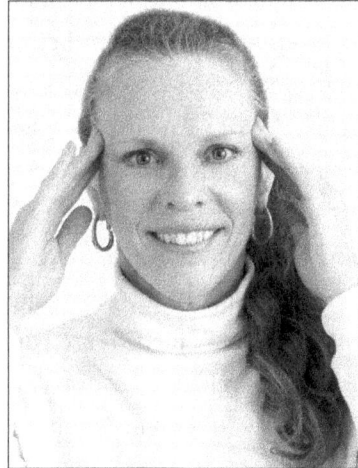

FIGURE 9.10
Massaging the temples.

Clenching and/or Grinding while Sleeping

You might think that while you are sleeping, your jaw and body relax totally. On the contrary, people often take their tension with them to sleep. In fact, some people clench or grind their teeth only at night. For improving general relaxation before sleeping, practice your Deep Relaxation tape as you lie in bed. Patients report to me on a regular basis that they feel more relaxed after practicing this tape than after a full night's sleep. This is a clear indication of how much tension people can take with them into their sleep.

If you have determined that you clench or grind while you are sleeping, it is important to program messages into your subconscious mind to break this pattern. This is quite simple to do. You may recall that when your mind is actively thinking your brain experiences beta waves, which are the fastest brain waves. While you are sleeping, your brain waves are the slowest, or delta. When you drift off to sleep and move from beta to delta, you will pass through alpha and theta brain-wave states as you become more and more deeply relaxed. We know from studies that the subconscious mind is most receptive to mental messages as you move into these slower brain-wave patterns. Therefore, it is most effective to program positive messages, or "positive affirmations," as you are drifting through alpha and theta brain-wave states.

At night while you are lying in bed before going to sleep, take a few deep, relaxing breaths and say to yourself, "My jaw is relaxed all through the night." Repeat this affirmation over and over as you are falling asleep. If your mind drifts off to other thoughts, gently bring it back to this affirmation. Repeat the affirmation slowly and with intention. Be sure your teeth are slightly apart and the tongue is relaxed down. Feel your jaw relaxing more and more as you repeat the affirmation.

Do this each night as you lie in bed before falling asleep. You might not see results immediately because it can take up to 30 days of consistent programming for an affirmation to be effective. Still, this positive, relaxing step before sleeping can ultimately help you release the tension leading to grinding and/or clenching, which in turn can help you to keep the muscle tension in your head at normal.

Psycho-Emotional Aspects of Jaw Tension

If you had to guess, why do you think you hold excess muscle tension in the jaw? Take some time to really think about the answer to this question. Is it due to repressed anger or frustration? Do you clench or tighten with physical pain? Are you holding back something that you would like to say to someone? Or, is this simply a place in your body where you hold stress?

It can be helpful to understand why you hold tension here. Sometimes just the awareness alone can help you begin to relax this part of your body. For example, if you now know that you clench when in physical pain or when stressed, you can be aware at those times to relax the jaw.

Remember, too, that sometimes there can be physical reasons for jaw problems. As I mentioned earlier, poor dental work or a motor vehicle accident can contribute to T.M.J. problems. However, in my experience when patients have tension in the T.M.J. area caused by a physical problem, they still are able to release the tension.

I once treated a 40-year-old woman named Tara who had suffered her whole life from debilitating migraines. Tara was born with one side of her jaw a half inch shorter than the other. Her doctor referred her to me for biofeedback training since her only other option was to have the jaw broken to make the two sides balanced, which she was understandably opposed to. When I attached the instruments up to measure the tension in her masseter muscles, I found that one side was at "normal' tension and the other side was 12 times normal. I had never seen such an extreme imbalance, and I noticed a thought going through my mind that said, "She will never be able to balance this out because of her physiology." Fortunately, I would never speak aloud such a limiting thought. Tara was, in fact, able to bring the readings into balance and to reach "normal tension" on both sides. Further, she brought both her muscle tension headaches and migraines under control. So, please don't use a physically based T.M.J. problem as an excuse for being unable to release jaw tension. If this woman could do it, you certainly can, too.

Practice

1. Cue dots – This week relax the jaw and affirm, "My jaw is calm and relaxed" every time you see a cue dot. Are you still noticing your dots, or is it time to change their color?

2. Jaw exercises – If possible, do the series of jaw exercises outlined in this lesson once or twice a day. If this is not possible, rotate the jaw exercises with the other exercises you are doing.

3. Pterygoid massage – Massage the pterygoid muscles two to three times a week.

4. Do the jaw and temple massage often.

5. Nighttime clenching or grinding – If you clench or grind while sleeping, remember to program the following affirmation into your subconscious mind: "My jaw is calm and relaxed all through the night."

6. Anger and frustration – If you discovered that you hold tension in your jaw area due to repressed anger or frustration (a

type of anger), there are several things you can do. First, there are many good books on anger. Some are quite practical and will teach you what you can do about anger. Look through several and see what you feel drawn to. A second option is to take a class in anger management. A third option is to see a psychotherapist or other professional to work on your anger issues.

Spend an entire week on this lesson before moving on to Lesson 10.

If you have continued to follow this program carefully, you will have begun seeing a significant reduction in the intensity and frequency of your stress induced symptoms by now. Your doctor has possibly reduced medications that are no longer necessary. This is a good time to take a look at your stress charts and acknowledge your improvement. *Do not be tempted to stop the program now.* You have a few more very important skills to learn.

5

Tap into the Power of Your Mind

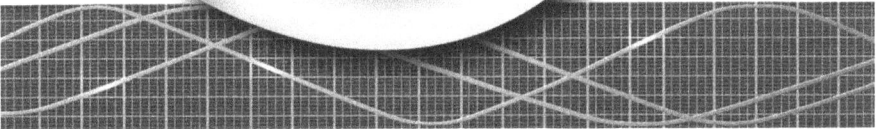

Lesson 10

Using Your Thoughts to Heal

How Your Thoughts Contribute to Your Stress Reaction

In order to gain control of your reaction to stress, you need to gain control of the tension in both your body *and* your mind. Any thought that causes you stress will lead to a number of physiological changes. Remember, every thought you have creates both a chemical change in the body and an electrical change in your nervous system. Your autonomic nervous system can shift from the parasympathetic to the sympathetic with a single thought.

Thoughts are so powerful that they create both physical and emotional reactions. In fact, all emotions come from either conscious or subconscious thoughts. Let me give you an example. Imagine you are on your way to a meeting and you get stuck in a traffic jam. You

133

might think, "This is terrible! This is awful! It's so unfair. I'm going to be late. What will they think?" Your emotional reaction as a result of this thinking would probably be anger and frustration. Your physical reaction might be increased muscle tension, short and shallow breathing, increased heart rate and rising blood pressure. You might even notice your hands and/or feet getting cold as the arteries constrict.

Now, imagine again that you are driving to an important meeting and you get stuck in a traffic jam. This time you think, "This is unfortunate, but there is nothing I can do to change the situation so I will give them a quick call to let them know I'll be late. Then, I might as well put on my favorite CD and listen to some good music. I think I will do some deep breathing and stretching to calm down even more." In this case, you would have chosen to feel in control emotionally and accepting of the situation. Physically, you might notice more relaxation in your body than before the traffic jam with your muscles relaxing, your breathing deepening, your heart rate slowing and your blood pressure going down.

What Is Self-Talk?

The nature of the mind is that it is a never-ending stream of thought. This stream of thought is sometimes called self-talk. You may not be aware of it, but you talk to yourself all the time in your thoughts. One of the most powerful tools for keeping your body in the parasympathetic nervous system, or shifting back to the parasympathetic from the sympathetic, is reframing your stressful self-talk. Since your moods, emotions and feelings are created and sustained by your self-talk, it stands to reason that if you alter the way you talk to yourself, you can change how you feel. Negative thoughts and their resulting emotions not only take the joy out of your life but also directly contribute to your physical and mental stress symptoms.

What Are Positive Affirmations?

Since thoughts have such powerful physical and emotional effects, it is important to be aware of and to *reframe* any stressful thoughts you might have. By reframing, we mean simply to change what you say to yourself. Imagine that your mind is like a computer. Your brain is the hardware, and the thoughts are the software. You were born with an unprogrammed mind. All the thoughts, ideas and beliefs were programmed into it. Some worked very well and served you. Some of the thoughts that were programmed early in your life may still support your life and health in a positive way today. Other thoughts, ideas and beliefs might cause you stress or anxiety. Those are the thoughts we want to reframe. We simply need to delete the stressful thoughts from the hard drive and replace them with what we call *positive affirmations*–that is, positive statements that we declare with feeling, power and belief. Working with positive affirmations is a very powerful way to calm the mind and the resulting emotions, thus creating a shift in your ANS to bring it back to homeostasis. Remember, homeostasis is where you need to keep your ANS to prevent physical and mental breakdowns from ocurring.

Examples of Positive Affirmations

Listed below are some examples of stressful thoughts (ST) that might pass through a person's mind followed by examples of positive affirmations (PA) that could be used instead for reprogramming. You may have many of these stressful thoughts yourself. Feel free to use any of these positive affirmations that are fitting for you. Additionally, you will later be learning how to make your own personal positive affirmations that are specific to your own life situations.

ST: "I never have enough money."
PA: "All my needs are taken care of in this moment."
 "Money comes to me easily and effortlessly."
 "I am grateful for the prosperity I have in my life."

ST: "I get so tense when I'm driving. I hate driving!"
PA: "I remember to breathe and relax when in the car."
 "I allow more than enough time to get to where I am going."

ST: "It's so unfair that I feel pain. I hate my body sometimes."
PA: "I am patient with my body as I move through my healing
 process."
 "I choose to be empowered; I am not a victim."
 "I listen to my body; the body doesn't lie."

ST: "I don't like my job at all, and I dread going to work
 each day."
PA: "I have the strength and courage to move out of my comfort
 zone and find a new job."
 "I am grateful for the experience and financial security my
 current job is giving me."

ST: "I get so tense at work."
PA: "I remember to breathe and relax while at work."
 "I relax no matter what the circumstances."

ST: "I don't like myself."

PA: "I let go of the judgment I place upon myself."

"It's okay to not be perfect."

"I remember to be kind, gentle and loving with myself."

ST: "I never have enough time to do what needs to get done."

PA: "Everything will get done in its own time; I can relax."

"I am in control of my time. I choose how I spend my time."

"I have enough time to do everything that is important to me."

ST: "I feel like I have to do everything."

PA: "I can say 'No' and it's okay."

"I don't have to take on everything."

ST: "I feel guilty if I take time to relax. I feel like I should be doing something."

PA: "It's okay to relax; I choose to take time out each day to relax."

"I relax for my health and well-being."

ST: "I know I won't be able to sleep tonight, and I will be groggy and irritable tomorrow." (Note: The sleep affirmations are the *only* affirmations that I suggest patients use even if the affirmations are not at all true for them. These can be helpful to program in even with the absence of truth.)

PA: "I fall asleep easily and effortlessly."

"I sleep peacefully all through the night."

"I wake up feeling refreshed and alert."

ST: "I'm afraid my financial future is not safe."

PA: "I do all that I can to ensure my financial future; I can relax."

"I trust that I am capable of taking care of my needs."

ST: "I hate it when I have negative emotions."
PA: "I accept and embrace all of my emotions."
    "I do not judge my emotions as good or bad."

ST: "I don't like my body."
PA: "I am grateful for how well my body has served me
      throughout my life."
     "I love and accept my body just as it is."

ST: "I worry about my children."
PA: "I choose to support my children with what they are going
     through rather than take on what they are going through."
     "I let my children experience their lives and feelings;
     I trust that they will be okay."

ST: "I worry about my grown children."
PA: "I let my children live their lives as they choose."
     "I let my children take responsibility for their choices and
     decisions."

ST: "I hate it when my body is in pain."
PA: "I remember to breathe and relax even when my body feels
     uncomfortable."
     "I am patient with my body as I bring it back into balance."

ST: "I feel so guilty."
PA: "I release my guilt. It serves no constructive purpose."
     "I replace the word 'should' with 'choose to' or 'want to.'"
     "I do not 'should' on myself!"

ST: "I'm stressed because of what other people think of me."

PA: "What other people think of me is none of my business."

"I am safe around people no matter what they are thinking. I can relax."

ST: "I just don't understand him/her."

PA: "I release my need to understand people and work to accept people as they are."

ST: "I feel like people walk all over me."

PA: "I stand up for myself and my rights."

"I am assertive. I stand up for what I need and want."

ST: "I feel so helpless and dependent when I am in pain."

PA: "I graciously accept when others choose to give to me."

"When I accept help, it does not take away from anybody else."

"I release my pride and become willing to accept help from others."

ST: "My mind just races out of control."

PA: "I am the master of my mind. I control my thoughts— they don't control me."

ST: "I hate to ask for support."

PA: "It is okay to ask for support."

"I attract people into my life who are supportive of me."

"I allow others to support me, and I relax with it."

ST: "That really shouldn't have happened to me."

PA: "I trust that I am always in the right place at the right time doing exactly the right thing."

"Everything is in perfect, divine order."

"I believe that everything happens for a reason and a purpose."

"I am capable of handling any challenge that comes my way."

ST: "I hate taking medications."

PA: "I am grateful for my medications."

"I am patient while I work to release the need for medications."

Making Your Own Personal Affirmations

There are five guidelines for writing your own personal positive affirmations.

1. Always state your affirmation in the present tense. For example, a poor affirmation is, "I will relax next month after my taxes are done." It would be better to say, "I breathe and relax in this moment" or "I choose to relax now."

2. Keep the affirmations short. You want both your conscious and subconscious mind to hear your affirmations. The subconscious mind can grasp short affirmations more easily. If you have an affirmation that seems like a long, run-on sentence, either shorten it or break it down into two affirmations.

3. Don't focus on the negative. For example, a poor affirmation is: "I am not a cigarette smoker." A good affirmation is, "I put only healthy things into my body."

4. Make your statements believable to yourself. They can work even if they are only a little bit believable. If it feels like a total lie, and there is no part of you that believes it, the affirmation will not work. For example, if your stressful thought is "I will never get rid of this anxiety" and you try to replace it with the thought "I don't have any anxiety" but this is not true, it simply will not work. A better affirmation would be, "I can learn to control my anxiety" or "I am now in the process of managing my anxiety."

5. Be specific when writing affirmations. A poor affirmation is, "My life is getting better" because "better" is a very vague word. A more specific affirmation is, "My body is healthier and stronger with each passing day."

Making your own affirmations involves a few steps. First, list areas of stress in your life without getting into detail at this point. For example, you might list finances, relationship with spouse, work, not having enough time, and so on.

Now, pick one of these areas of stress and list all the thoughts you have related to this area that cause you stress. For example, under finances, you might write, "I never have enough money." Remember to stick to writing only the thoughts and not the emotions or body sensations. This is because using positive affirmations to work with thoughts and beliefs works at a deeper level than working with emotions or body sensations. This work on thoughts will begin to resolve the negative emotions and physical reactions you have to the thought.

For each thought, write at least one positive affirmation following the five guidelines listed above. Repeat this process with each area of stress you listed, fully exhausting the thoughts you have in that category. Try not to judge yourself or your thoughts as you do this exercise.

Repetition is important when working with positive affirmations. Your old thoughts and beliefs will come back into your mind because they are there out of habit. It is going to take some conscious work to change these habitual thought patterns. Psychologists say it can take 30 days to change an old thought and create a new positive *belief*, which is a thought that you accept as truth. It is important that you work with your new thoughts daily. Use your positive affirmation notebook, the tape, the cue dots, and catching yourself on the spot to begin reframing your negative thoughts into positive thoughts that will evolve into positive beliefs over time.

Practice

1. Make your own personal positive affirmations using the guidelines in this lesson.

2. Record your personal positive affirmations on tape. Speak slowly, clearly and with intention as you record your affirmations. You can use relaxing music in the background if you like. Read each affirmation at least two times pausing after each one you read. The first time you read the affirmation, speak from the first person (I…). Then speak the affirmation from the second person (You…). Finally, speak the affirmation with your name, if you like (Kate…). This way, your subconscious is hearing it from several different perspectives. For example, "I love and accept my body just as it is…You love and accept your body just as it is…Kate loves and accepts her body just as it is."

As with the body/mind relaxation tape and the imagery tape, the most powerful time to listen to this tape is while you are falling asleep or waking up. With the addition of this affirmation tape, you will have three tapes that you can rotate.

3. Create a positive affirmation notebook. Every time you experience stress, look at the thoughts that created the stress and write them down. You might become aware of the emotion first. If you notice you feel frustration, anger, anxiety, jealousy, insecurity or any stressful emotion, look a little deeper to discover the thought(s) that created that emotion. Then write the thought(s) down on one side of the notebook. On the other side, write one or more positive affirmations that you can use to replace the stressful thought.

4. Pick one positive affirmation each day that you would like to work with. Every time you see a cue dot, take a deep breathe and say the affirmation to yourself.

5. Catch your negative self-talk on the spot. If you notice a negative or stressful thought, see if you can delete it immediately and replace it with a positive affirmation that will leave you feeling calm and relaxed.

Spend one full week on this lesson. If it feels like that is not enough time, spend up to two weeks before moving on to the next lesson. Be sure to give yourself sufficient time to start integrating this new thinking into your life. Working with changing the mind can be the hardest work for some people. Be patient and remember that you are just playing with thoughts, and thoughts can be changed. Have fun with it!

Increase Your Circulation

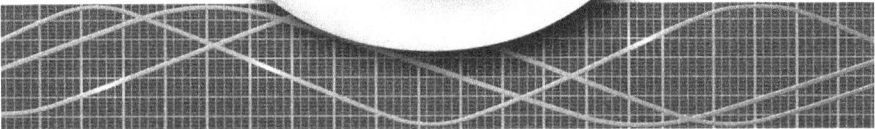

Dilating Your Arteries for Deeper Relaxation

Why You Need to Increase Your Circulation

You may recall that one of the many ways your body responds to stress is by constricting the smooth muscles that surround the arteries. Familiarize yourself with the anatomy of the arteries by looking at the illustration in fig. 11.1. During the fight-or-flight response, your body automatically constricts blood flow. That way, if you were to be attacked or cut, you would bleed less. Remember, this is one way the body protects itself. The problem, as mentioned earlier, is that your body responds with this automatic physiological reaction not only during a physical threat, but also during times of psychological stress. And because most of us experience lots of psychological stress in our fast-paced world, our bodies can suffer physical consequences, such as migraine headaches or high blood pressure, from this restriction of blood flow.

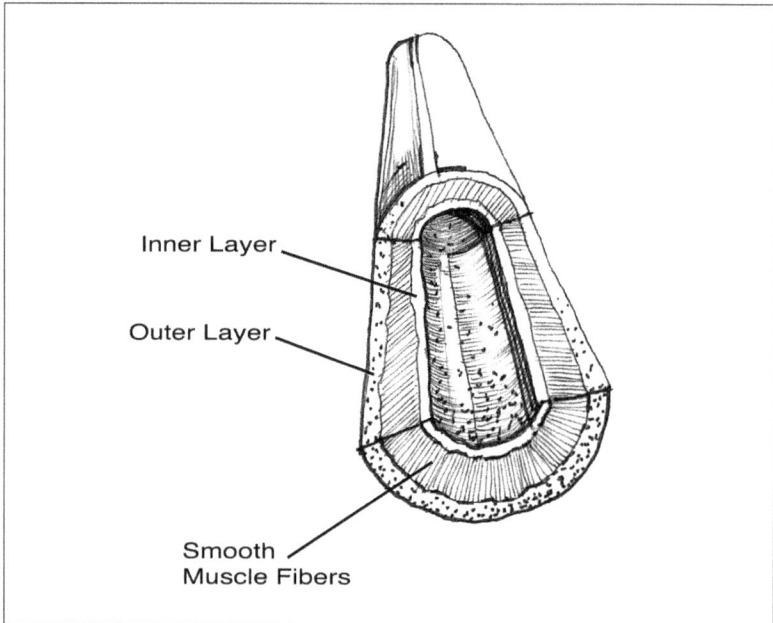

FIGURE 11.1—The smooth muscles make up the bulk of the artery.

People who hold stress in their vascular system usually have a tendency towards cold hands and feet. If you are taking medications for hypertension or migraines it is likely they are vaso-dilators. In other words, the medications keep your arteries dilated instead of doing that job for yourself. Stay on your medications until your doctor instructs you otherwise. And, do the temperature training anyway. You will be starting with a higher surface skin temperature than you would if you were not on the medications and that is okay. Sometimes people experience cold hands and feet when they are stressed but do not develop vascular diseases. Temperature training is another skill that is beneficial for everyone to learn in order to balance the nervous system.

Do you remember the "mood rings" of the 1960s? Did you ever think about how they worked? Simply put, the rings responded to the temperature of your hands, turning a particular color depending upon the temperature. If you were relaxed and the blood was flowing freely to your hands, your surface skin temperature would be warmer, and the ring would show a color supposedly indicating that you were in a "good mood." If the temperature of your hands was cooler due to constricted arteries, the ring's inventors knew this could indicate that you were experiencing stress and labeled this a "bad mood." The mood rings were actually a simplistic form of biofeedback, or biological feedback—they would give feedback about what was going on in your body.

All of the previous lessons have begun to bring your nervous system into balance, or homeostasis. Chances are you have already started to increase your circulation with the practice of the new skills you have been learning. You are probably already experiencing a dramatic reduction in the number and intensity of your stress related symptoms. Perhaps they are even completely gone. But even if they are gone, do this lesson anyway. This lesson is the icing on the cake, teaching you regulation of one very important physiological element.

How to Increase Your Circulation

In biofeedback, your circulation is measured simply by taking the temperature on the surface of your skin. If the smooth muscles around the arteries are relaxed and the blood is flowing freely, you will have a temperature of 93 degrees or higher on the surface of your skin. Of course, internally, your temperature is approximately 98.6 degrees.

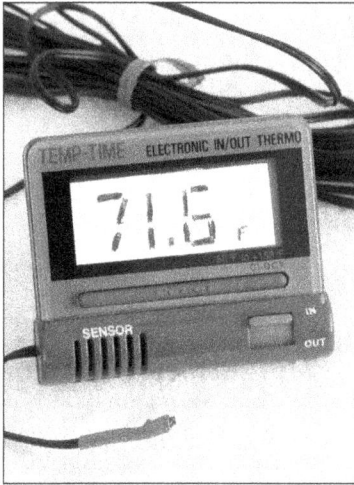

FIGURE 11.2

SST training unit

We start by measuring the temperature on your fingertips. I frequently see people with migraines who initially have a temperature in the low 80s or even the high 70s on the surface of their fingertips. This indicates a great deal of constriction in the arteries. They need to learn how to maintain their surface skin temperature (SST) at 93 degrees or higher to completely eliminate their migraines.

Since you have already been practicing numerous skills for bringing the nervous system into balance as you have worked through this program, it is likely that your SST has been going up over the last weeks or months. You may be starting with an SST in the high 80s or low 90s as you begin this lesson due to the work you have already done. *Still, it is essential that you do this lesson anyway!*

You will need a simple digital thermometer with a wire extension (called a *thermistor*) to measure your progress with the temperature training (fig. 11.2). It is important to have an instrument that goes up in increments of one-tenth of a degree at a time (0.1). This sensitivity is necessary to get good feedback of your progress. SST measurement units are available at the website listed at the bottom of this page. These units will have the sensitivity that you need in order to do temperature training.

If you do not already have your temperature unit but you are ready to get started on this lesson, you can begin without the unit.

Many people can feel the warmth increasing in their hands and feet. Some people are very in tune with their bodies and don't even need the feedback from an instrument. You certainly can start practicing hand and foot warming before you have your unit.

Chemical stimulants and vasoconstrictors will work against you in temperature training. Hopefully, early on in the program you eliminated caffeine and nicotine completely from your diet if you hold stress in your vascular system. Caffeine and nicotine will make it difficult, if not impossible, for you to get your SST above 93 degrees. If you have either of these substances left in your diet, now is a great time to eliminate them completely.

Temperature Training

You are now ready to begin temperature training. Make sure the room you are training in is between 70 and 74 degrees. If you came in from the outdoors and it was hotter or colder than this outside, wait for 15 minutes before beginning temperature training.

Find a comfortable place to sit down; a recliner is perfect, but any comfortable location will do. Wear loose, comfortable clothing. Make sure you will not have any distractions or interruptions. Turn off your phone.

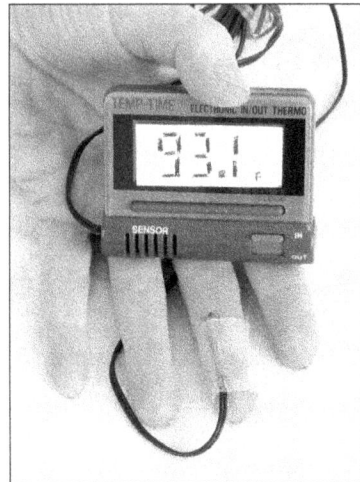

FIGURE 11.3
Attaching thermistor to fingertip.

Some people prefer to have soothing music in the background while others prefer to practice in silence.

Now, using medical tape, attach the last inch of the thermistor to the pad of one of your fingertips (fig. 11.3). You might want to start with your right hand if you are right-handed or your left hand if you are left-handed. *Do not tape over the little glass ball at the very end of the thermistor.*

Next, you need to get your "baseline" temperature. The baseline temperature is where the temperature levels off before you begin practicing hand warming. When you attach the thermistor to your finger, it will begin to move up from the room temperature to your baseline SST. The temperature usually levels off within two minutes, but this is not always the case. Consider the temperature level when it has stayed consistent for approximately half a minute. When it levels off, record this temperature to the nearest tenth of a degree.

Now you will practice dilating your arteries and warming your hands for five to ten minutes. You can do this either with your eyes open or closed. Many people find that it is easier to focus on the internal workings of their body with their eyes closed. However, some people do better with their eyes open so that they can watch the feedback on the monitor. Do what works best for you. You will be given some tips on ways to warm your hands or feet in the following section.

After you have worked on warming your hands for at least five minutes, look at your temperature unit and write down your "end temperature," or your temperature after training. Then write down whether you have gone up or down and by how much. For example, if your baseline temperature was 89.0 degrees and your temperature after training was 91.5 degrees, write down +2.5 degrees. Keep a chart of your temperature training to track your progress.

You need to *generalize* this training in order for it to be effective in increasing your body's circulation. In other words, if you were to work on warming your right hand only, you wouldn't necessarily increase the circulation throughout your whole body. Instead, you would likely only warm your right hand with this approach. That is why you need to train both hands and both feet. Master the hand warming first before moving on to the feet. Ultimately, you will need to be able to maintain the SST of both hands and both feet at 93 degrees or higher.

When you start training both your hands and feet, write down which you are working on each day. For example, LH for left hand, RF for right foot, etc. Notice whether it is easier to warm your hands or your feet. Notice whether one side of your body has a lower temperature than the other.

Date	Room	Baseline	End temp.	Hand/Foot	Change
4/11	73	87.1	91.3	R.H.	+4.2
4/12	71	89.4	90.9	L.H.	+1.5

FIGURE 11.4—Sample temperature training chart.

Charting Your Progress

You will need to create a chart to track your progress with raising your SST. It should include date of practice, the room temperature, your baseline temperature, your end temperature, which hand or foot you were training and the amount your SST went up or down while training. See a sample chart in fig. 11.4. If you have *The Stress Mess Workbook*, you will find a temperature training chart in there that you can copy and use.

Being Successful at Regulating Your Blood Flow

You can regulate blood flow in your body by using the power of your mind, imagination, breathing and general relaxation. When you are able to warm both hands and both feet, you are increasing the circulation in your entire body. Skills you've already developed in this program will help you reach that point:

1. Deep, slow diaphragmatic breathing helps to dilate the arteries. Try doing ten minutes of this breathing with your temperature unit hooked up and see what happens!

2. Use your imagination. Visualize the arteries dilating. You don't need to know where the arteries are for this to work. Or, imagine you are holding your hands over an open campfire and you are feeling the warmth…or perhaps you are putting your hands into a dishpan of warm water…or you are walking barefoot on the beach and feeling the warmth of the sand on your feet. Create the feeling of warmth in your body. Use whatever image comes to you when you think of warmth in your body.

3. Use affirmations. This is very effective for people who are more auditory than visual or kinesthetic. Some examples of messages you might use are, "My arms and hands are warm" or "My legs and feet are relaxed and warm." Repeat the mental messages and notice whether you can feel the warming.

4. Sometimes people can warm their hands or feet just by looking at the feedback on the monitor and imagining the temperature going up.

For some people temperature training comes easily, and for others it is the most difficult part of the training. Do not be discouraged if at first you do not succeed. Be patient and stick with it. You will get it! If at first your temperature is going down during the training instead of going up, ask yourself if you are trying too hard. If you are stressing to get your temperature up, you will get just the opposite result.

I had one migraine patient named Andrea whose temperature kept dropping for the first three sessions we worked on blood flow. Finally, during the third session I said to her, "If you had to guess, why do you think this is happening?" Andrea immediately blurted out, "Because this is the most important part of the training and I have to get it right!" Once that answer came out of her mouth, she laughed and realized what she had been doing. Her temperature immediately started going up, and Andrea never had a problem with warming her hands again.

Practice

1. Make a charting system to track your progress with raising your SST.

2. Practice temperature training once or twice daily, but do so for no more than five or ten minutes at a time. If you work too long or try to do too much in one session, you will lose focus and possibly get frustrated, which will cause your temperature to drop as you become stressed.

3. Are you staying on track with deep breathing, the relaxation, imagery and positive affirmation tapes, responding to your cue dots, relaxing specific muscles and stopping/reframing stressful thoughts?

You probably have your stress symptoms significantly under control at this point. Still, it is important to continue to practice temperature training and the other skills previously learned. Do not be tempted to stop even if your symptoms are fully under control. If they are not yet fully under control, continue to practice and know that for some people it takes longer to change these internal habits. Be patient with yourself and your body as you perfect and master the skills presented in this program.

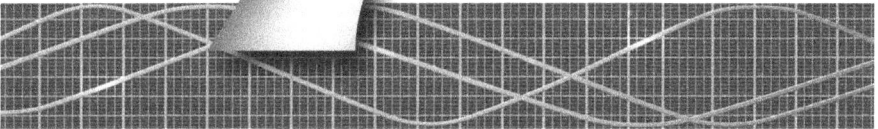

7

Stay on Track

12

Living
Beyond the Stress Mess

Congratulations!

Congratulations! Celebrate! You are at the end of the beginning! If you have followed this program very carefully, you are probably no longer suffering from your stress-related symptoms. You might think you no longer need to practice the skills you've learned here since your symptoms are now gone. But it was practicing the skills that led you to become healthy, and continuing to practice these skills will keep you healthy. You have worked for at least a few months by now to create new habits, and you have created a "new normal" level of tension in your body and your mind. The hard work is already done. Now you simply need to maintain your nervous system in homeostasis.

You will have integrated many of the stress reduction techniques you have learned in this program into your life by now so that they have become automatic. You have created some good new habits. However, as you know, old habits are hard to break; they tend to creep back into our lives when we are not paying attention. It is important at this point to decide what you will do so that you can continue to enjoy being symptom-free. Make a commitment to yourself and your support person (if you have one) about what you will do to stay symptom-free. Speak it aloud and affirm it with passion and intention.

You may have noticed as you moved through the lessons that some of your old habits were harder to break than others. Think about which habits were harder to let go of–those will be the habits requiring the most attention and the most focus in the future. For example, did you find it hard to replace old stressful thoughts with new positive ones? Did you find it hard to cut caffeine out of your diet? Did you find it hard to do the relaxation tape of the body and mind? Make a written note of the parts of this training that were the hardest for you so that you can remind yourself to continue to practice and be vigilant in these areas.

Excuses for Getting off Track

If you do get off track and find yourself returning to old habits, become aware of what your mind is saying to you about your new practice. It might say something like, "I'm not feeling stressed so I don't need to practice today," or "I'm too busy today; I just don't have the time to practice," or "Missing one day won't hurt." Our minds can come up with some very seductive excuses!

If you choose to stay symptom-free, it will be important to catch the thoughts that can stop you from staying on track. Then reframe each thought so that it will serve you and keep you on track. For example, you could reframe the thought, "I'm too busy today; I just don't have the time to practice," into "I'm very busy today, so I am only going to spend ten minutes doing my shoulder exercises." Or you could reframe the thought, "I'm not feeling stressed so I don't need to practice today," to say "I'm not feeling stressed today and I choose to do my relaxation exercises anyway." This way, you will be acknowledging the thought but giving it a positive spin in order to stay on track.

Do something every single day to release the stress from your body and mind. Let daily practice be your new habit and commitment to living free of stress symptoms.

Sometimes people believe that they have to do all of their work before they have a right to relax. If you believe that, think about what positive affirmations you can use to support yourself in staying on track. For example, "My health is the most important thing. I relax for my health and well-being." It might help to remind yourself that the amount of time that it takes to do these exercises is minute in comparison to the amount of time you expend on having stress symptoms. Consider also the impact your symptoms have on your social life, finances, and energy. And besides, relaxation is a whole lot more fun!

Most people begin to experience more energy as a result of practicing stress reduction exercises such as those presented in this book. They become calmer and more positive, productive and focused. Nervous energy and anxiety no longer spur most of their actions. The feeling of spinning their wheels disappears as relaxation moves in. So, if you are one of those people who think you would be less productive while relaxed, understand that just the opposite is true.

If you find that you continue to make excuses and don't take control of your stress, it will be time to look at what you are getting out of that behavior. You now know that you can control your symptoms, and you also know how to do so. If you choose not to, you might want to look at why you don't want to get rid of your symptoms. You may not consciously be aware of what you are getting out of continuing to have such symptoms. However, there is a very good chance that your symptoms provide you with what is known as a "secondary gain" or benefit of some sort. For example, perhaps your backache gets you out of some social situation you want to avoid. With your back pain you have a perfectly good excuse for not participating. Maybe you get a lot of attention when you are in pain, or perhaps this is how you get some alone time. Be honest with yourself about the possibility that you are getting some secondary gain from having symptoms even if they truly make you suffer as well.

In my experience, only an extremely small percentage of people with stress symptoms get off track once their stress is managed. If you occasionally get a little bit off track, don't beat yourself up. Simply get back on track as soon as you can. Often when people go on vacation or travel, they get out of their routines. If this happens to you, it might be helpful to create a positive affirmation such as, "I am back on track and I do the best I can."

I find that most people with chronic pain or headaches are highly motivated and generally do stay on track. They rarely make up excuses in my experience. Pain can be a big motivator for a person to take control of their nervous system.

Support Is Available

It was suggested very early in this program that you find a "support partner" if you wanted support. You may have gone through this program without support from anyone else. Some people do fine on their own while others are more successful with support. If you did the program alone and found it difficult, you might want to rethink the idea of getting a support partner now.

If you feel as if you would benefit from additional support in reducing the stress in your body and mind, you might consider consulting a professional. If you are interested in one-on-one sessions, I would suggest that you learn relaxation skills from a certified biofeedback therapist in your area. Make sure this professional is certified by the Biofeedback Certification Institute of America (BCIA). This is the only legitimate biofeedback certification. Go to www.BCIA.org to learn more.

Professional coaching and support are also available from the author of this book. You will find information about these services at NaturallyStressFree.com. I will be happy to evaluate your needs and set up phone sessions to support you. Seminars and keynotes are also available through Naturally Stress Free.

Classes are another way to stay on track or to renew your commitment. Classes in stress reduction are often available through continuing education programs, hospitals and company health plans. A gentle yoga class can help enormously to calm the body and still the mind. To find one that works for you, sample a few classes with various styles and different teachers. There are as many different styles as there are teachers, so find a style and teacher you will enjoy.

Frequently Asked Questions

I have found that many patients have the same questions about this program. I have included several of these questions here with responses that I hope will meet the individual needs of most readers.

How effective is this program?

Nearly all the patients I have worked with have either completely eliminated their symptoms or dramatically reduced the intensity of their symptoms. I am happy to be able to report that this program has been effective with over 90 percent of the people with which I have worked. Granted, the people who came to me were ready to conquer their stress or they would not have come. They were motivated and followed the program carefully. I have received numerous emails and phone calls from around the country where people have reported bringing their headaches under control by following this program which was first presented in the book *Migraines Be Gone.*

However, there was an instance where a client did not have success, and it is worth telling the story. A woman named Cynthia came to me for treatment of her migraines. During the first session I asked her when her migraines started. She reported that they began when her husband was killed suddenly several years earlier. Her life crumbled and fell apart. Cynthia said that she had the "perfect life" before that tragedy, and it was all shattered. Her whole identity was tied up with this man, his profession and role in the community and her role as his wife. She loved the role she played. When he was killed, she not only lost her husband, she felt that she also lost her "perfect life," her role and her identity.

Eight years had passed since the death of her first husband when Cynthia came to work with me, and she had remarried during that period. Interestingly, several times in our sessions she referred to her current husband by her former husband's name. She would catch what she said and look surprised. After several sessions there was absolutely no improvement with the number or intensity of headaches she was having. At that point I suggested that she see a professional who specialized in trauma issues. Cynthia was not receptive to the idea but agreed that we had done all we could together.

In my experience people can generally control their symptoms if they are dedicated, practice and master the skills and stay on track. If you have issues of unresolved trauma, as in the case above, you may need to address those issues first. Trauma throws the autonomic nervous system into dramatic swings between the SNS and the PNS. Trauma would include such things as experiencing war, rape, violence, extreme loss, and even surgery for some people.

Let's look at irritable bowel syndrome (IBS) with regards to trauma and the ANS. If the ANS swings far into the SNS, or fight or flight response, digestion shuts down causing constipation. Then the nervous system wants to come back to homeostasis, or balance, but now it swings too deep into the PSN as it strives to achieve balance. Then diarrhea is the result. The swings in the nervous system with trauma are much more pronounced than with more normal stressors.

With the major changes that are now occurring on the planet, we are likely to see more trauma on a massive scale. For example, think about the victims of Katrina who lost everything. Many lost not only their homes, jobs, income source, familiar surroundings, and friends by being dislocated, but some also lost loved ones who died in this tragedy. This amount of change and loss is very traumatic. It is far beyond having one loss or change to deal with. And, this trauma affected thousands of people. If our nervous systems are in balance, or homeostasis, we will have more resiliency when faced with trauma. If you train your nervous system now you will be better prepared to meet the global challenges and changes we face.

Do I have to do these exercises forever?

You can monitor your body to see how long you will need to stay on track with a structured program. Some people integrate these exercises and skills into their lives and find value in using them long after they have stopped having symptoms. Maintaining normal tension becomes such a habit that they don't have to think about formally doing the activities. They simply have created new habits. However, if you stop doing the program in a structured way and your symptoms return, you will know that you have not fully integrated the skills into your life. You will have moved back up to a level of high stress in the nervous system. If this happens, simply return to a more structured way of practicing.

How long will the results of this program last?

I have frequently met former patients years after they did this training who have told me their symptoms have been completely eliminated since doing the program or have remained dramatically reduced. The ones who have admitted that some symptoms have crept back into their lives have also admitted that they have gotten off track from the program. However, even these patients reported that their symptoms have not been nearly as bad as before the training. Most of the patients I have talked with after the training say that they still use the CDs and do the exercises because they enjoy it.

In Conclusion...

Congratulations for choosing to embark on this empowering journey. Your ability to manage your nervous system and heal your stress related physical and mental symptoms has tremendous power. Patients often report that once they have conquered their symptoms, they feel like they can conquer anything. My wish for you is that you continue to be the master of your body-mind and that you enjoy a pain-free and healthy life as you learn how to live *beyond* the stress mess.

Index

WIN PRIZES FOR SHARING YOUR STORIES AND YOUR FEEDBACK!

We would love to hear from you!
Please write us at the web site listed at
the bottom of this page and let us know...

- What were your results?

- Is there anything in the program that you felt could be improved in any way?

- What part(s) of the training were most powerful for you?

- What part(s) were the easiest and the most difficult?

- How long did you work on the program before you started seeing results?

- How long was it before the symptoms were totally under control?

- How has this program changed your life?

- How often did you have your symptoms before doing this program?

- If you have any stress symptoms remaining, how often do you get them now? What was the intensity level of the symptoms before and after the program?

Tell us whatever you like ... we love hearing your stories.

As a "thank you" for your feedback you will be entered into a semi-annual drawing where you could win prizes ranging from CDs to a free week-long retreat!

Thank you for your feedback and stories,
Kelsie Kenefick

Products and Services
to Support Your Well-Being

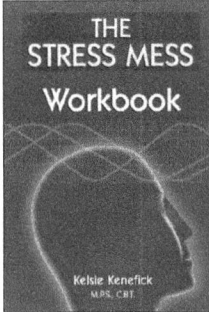

The Stress Mess Workbook

The Stress Mess Workbook contains all of the charts and worksheets necessary to track your progress. Additionally, there are worksheets included to support you in creating new habits and integrating the skills into your life. The book is available in hard copy or e-book.

Calming Your Body / Stilling Your Mind CD

Learn to bring your autonomic nervous system to a place of balance by practicing with the guidance of this CD. Calming nature sounds in the background aid in your relaxation.

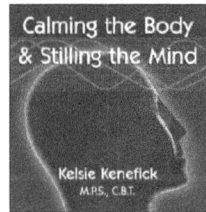

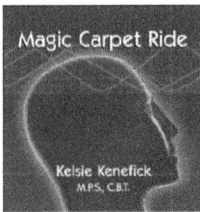

Magic Carpet Ride CD

Take a relaxing vacation without ever leaving your living room! Using the power of visualization you can learn how to travel anywhere you wish to go on your magic carpet. Calming nature sounds in the background aid in deepening your journey.

Stress Be Gone Exercises - DVD

Relax and practice your exercises with visual and verbal guidance. All of the shoulder, neck, jaw and eye exercises presented in this book are included in this DVD.

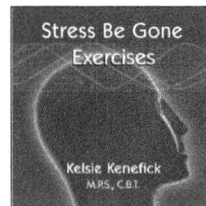

For more information go to
NaturallyStressFree.com

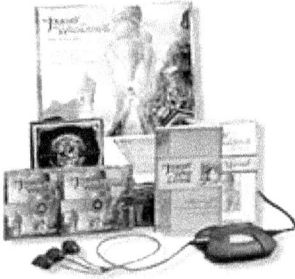

The Wild Divine – the first "inner-active" computer adventure!

Using biofeedback play over 40 games in this magical castle setting. You control the games by controlling your physiology! It is an entertaining and effective way to calm your body, still your mind, and improve your health.

Skin Temperature Biofeedback Unit

Learn to control your blood flow and circulation with this unit. The more you relax the warmer your hands and feet will become! This unit is especially good for anyone with migraine headaches, high blood pressure, or any vascular disorder…and is great for anyone wishing to learn how to control their physiological reaction to stress.

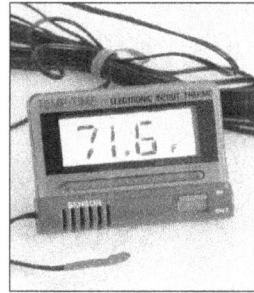

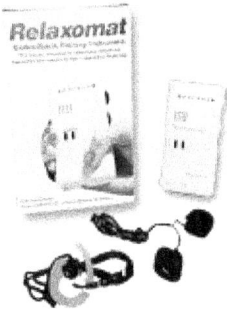

GSR biofeedback unit – Relaxomat

Galvanic skin response (GSR) measures sweat gland activity. Sweat gland activity can change instantly with just a thought so this is a very fun unit to work with! Relaxomat has both visual and auditory feedback. External finger electrodes and earphone included. Great for anyone interested in learning relaxation training!

The solution for computer-use discomfort

Stress Away Software – If your computer is a pain in the neck, Stress Away is for you!

This is an extremely effective program for preventing/reducing repetitive strain disorders caused by computer use. Throughout the day a guide will appear on your computer at regular intervals. The guide will lead you through a 30 second exercise to eliminate tension in your neck, head, wrists, shoulders or eyes. Increase your productivity by decreasing pain, discomfort, and fatigue. For Mac and PC.

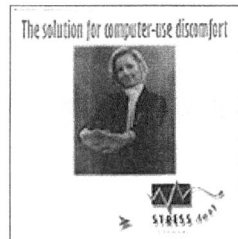

For more information go to NaturallyStressFree.com

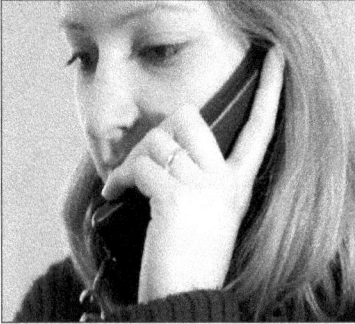

Phone Consultations

Do you have questions about any of the skills presented in this book? Do you need support with staying on track? The author of this book is available for phone consultations. Visit the web site listed at the bottom of this page and click on the "consultations" button for further information.

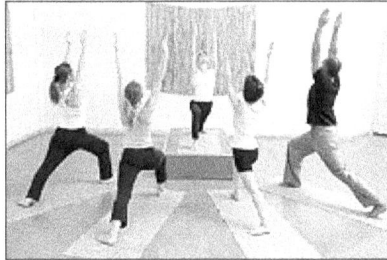

Keynotes, Seminars, and Retreats

Kelsie Kenefick is a Certified Seminar Trainer (C.S.T. – Peak Potentials) who uses accelerated learning techniques. Your group will learn a lot, will remember what they learn, and will have fun doing it! Kelsie has presented this work in school districts, hospitals, government organizations, and corporations. Book Kelsie today... money back guarantee!

Retreats are residential and are a time for you to completely focus on yourself and your well being as you learn how to control your stress reaction. They are typically held in the Colorado Rocky Mountains where you will learn the skills amidst spectacular views, clean air, and healing mineral hot springs nearby. Alternatively, they can be held at a location of your choice. Individual and group retreats are available.

For more information go to
NaturallyStressFree.com

www.ingramcontent.com/pod-product-compliance
Lightning Source LLC
Chambersburg PA
CBHW072235270326
41930CB00010B/2140